ANTI-INFLAMM
COOKBOOK
FOR BEGINNERS

MW00872840

Master 1500 Days of Easy, Quick and Delicious Recipes to Alleviate Chronic Pain, Boost Immunity, and Nourish Your Body
35-Days Meal Plan Included

Isabel Meadowcroft

© **Copyright 2023 by Isabel Meadowcroft - All rights reserved.**

The following book is provided below with the aim of delivering information that is as precise and dependable as possible. However, purchasing this book implies an acknowledgment that both the publisher and the author are not experts in the discussed topics, and any recommendations or suggestions contained herein are solely for entertainment purposes. It is advised that professionals be consulted as needed before acting on any endorsed actions.

This statement is considered fair and valid by both the American Bar Association and the Committee of Publishers Association, and it holds legal binding throughout the United States.

Moreover, any transmission, duplication, or reproduction of this work, including specific information, will be deemed an illegal act, regardless of whether it is done electronically or in print. This includes creating secondary or tertiary copies of the work or recorded copies, which are only allowed with the express written consent from the Publisher. All additional rights are reserved.

The information in the following pages is generally considered to be a truthful and accurate account of facts. As such, any negligence, use, or misuse of the information by the reader will result in actions falling solely under their responsibility. There are no scenarios in which the publisher or the original author can be held liable for any difficulties or damages that may occur after undertaking the information described herein.

Additionally, the information in the following pages is intended solely for informational purposes and should be considered as such. As fitting its nature, it is presented without assurance regarding its prolonged validity or interim quality. Mention of trademarks is done without written consent and should not be construed as an endorsement from the trademark holder.

TABLE OF CONTENTS

Lean and Flavorful Poultry Recipes 49

Sides and Appetizers: Tasty and Healthy Bites 61

Soups Recipes for All Seasons 71

Healthy Desserts Recipes 81

5-Week Meal Plan: Your Roadmap to Success 91

Conclusion 95

A Special Thank You 97

INTRODUCTION

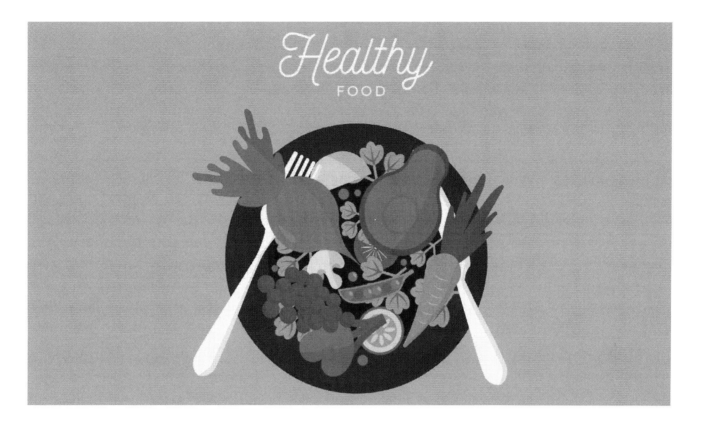

A WARM AND EMPATHETIC INTRODUCTION, ACKNOWLEDGING THE CHALLENGES AND ASPIRATIONS OF BEGINNING AN ANTI-INFLAMMATORY LIFESTYLE.

Embarking on the journey to a more vibrant, pain-free life can often feel like standing at the edge of a forest—lush with mystery, promise, and a fair share of uncertainties. As you stand there, you might be holding the weight of past diets, health regimens, and countless hours scouring the web for a reliable path through the dense thicket of wellness advice. I want you to know that I understand this undertaking is no small feat, and it marks the start of something incredibly meaningful.

You're not just changing what's on your plate; you're reshaping your daily rituals, redefining grocery lists, and perhaps most importantly, you're rekindling hope for more healthful, exuberant days ahead. I have witnessed this shift's power—from nagging discomfort fading like the last stars of dawn to newfound energy that courses through you like a springtime river. These are not mere possibilities; they are the destinations waiting along the road of the anti-inflammatory lifestyle.

Where conventional paths have left many feeling stranded in a cycle of medications and temporary fixes, the anti-inflammatory diet stands as a beacon, promising relief through nature's own pantry. It understands the language of your body, employing foods that silence the alarms of inflammation, the root of so much chronic pain and a myriad of health woes. It's a diet bunking the age-old adage—"You are what you eat," turning every meal into a dialogue with your body, fostering a nurturing conversation of healing and health.

But know this: it's perfectly human to harbor a trove of questions and uncertainties. Will these recipes fit the billow of my busy schedule? Can I actually savor meals without the ingredients I've come to love—indeed, rely on—over the years? And, nestled further within, the whisper of an even more fundamental question: Is the road ahead too steep for me?

First, let me ease those furrowed brows with assurance. The paths of change are well-trodden and the way, though new to you, is lined with the guideposts and helpful hints I've carefully laid out in this cookbook. Fear not the undertaking, nor the time it may require. Picture instead the mornings free of stiffness, the afternoons devoid of weariness, and the joyful reunions with your own vitality.

As we navigate this new landscape together, there will be discoveries—ingredients that you've passed by on supermarket aisles will now greet you like old friends, vegetables and spices will come together in delightful harmony you never thought possible. You'll redefine 'quick meals', no longer synonymous with takeouts or processed foods, but with vibrant, nourishing feasts that invigorate rather than inhibit.

I also appreciate the practicalities. You're balancing a crystalline vision of health with the gritty realities of day-to-day life—managing the demands of your roles as professionals, caretakers, educators, and more. Convenience cannot merely be a luxury—it's a necessity. Thus, each recipe within this book has been crafted with an eye for the clock and an understanding of bustling schedules. They are not only palatable to your taste buds but to your calendar as well.

And for the beginners among you simmering with apprehension over your nascent culinary skills, let me extend a compassionate hand. Cooking, like any art, begins with single, simple strokes—each additional layer adding depth, texture, and confidence. This book endeavors to be your companion in the kitchen, a gentle guide simmering alongside you as you stir, blend, and season your way to fluency in the language of anti-inflammatory cuisine.

Let's also talk brass tacks—budget. The cost of a healthful life shouldn't demand from you a king's ransom. I believe in the empowerment found in affordability, so while you may encounter ingredients that are new and perhaps exotic, know that this journey is tailored to be as accessible as it is enriching. You'll find that your investment in wholesome foods will yield dividends in the currency of health—a valuable exchange if there ever was one.

To the families poised to partake in this transition, your love for your kin is the secret ingredient that will make these recipes resonate beyond your own plate. The turn toward nutritious meals doesn't have to be a solo adventure; it's a shared feast of well-being that even the youngest of palates can enjoy with relish. And these pages are littered with tips to ensure those first bites turn into lifelong habits for everyone gathered at your table.

In the information-flooded world where the next best diet vies for your attention, the pull to surrender to inertia can be powerful. But this is not just another diet. It's an awakening to a lifestyle that honors your body's needs, preferences, and perhaps most critically, its cries for help. It's a patient and persistent pursuit of wellness.

Wave aside the concerns that the flavors of health will be muted compared to your current fare. These recipes are a testament—wholesome can also be hearty, nourishing can dazzle the tastebuds, and healthy food can be banquet-worthy. Together, we will craft meals that don't simply nourish—they celebrate every bite as a step toward a more vibrant you.

So, with a promise of support, a sprinkle of patience, and a steady pour of encouragement, let's turn this page and take the first steps. Welcome to a kitchen where every ingredient is a friend, every meal a milestone, and the end result is nothing less than a delicious revelation of health.

DISCOVERING THE POWER OF ANTI-INFLAMMATORY FOODS

In the bustling lanes of our daily lives, a silent epidemic spreads, largely unnoticed until it taps on our shoulders with aches and pains that turn chronic, immune systems that falter under pressure, and a fog of fatigue that dims the very vibrancy of our existence. But there's hope, a beacon of gentle, healing light in the embracing warmth of your own kitchen: the power of anti-inflammatory foods.

What exactly does inflammation mean for our bodies? Imagine a busy city street, traffic flowing smoothly, all is well. Now picture a car accident — nothing catastrophic, but suddenly, the order is disrupted. Police arrive, an ambulance, maybe a tow truck — all good and necessary responders, much like our body's immune system reacting to unwelcome invaders or injuries. However, if these responders never leave, if the disruption becomes the norm, the street turns into a constant site of stress and chaos. Chronic inflammation is much like this — when our immune system's response lingers incessantly, it begins to wear us down from the inside.

But just as traffic can be managed and streets cleared, so too can our bodies find a reprieve. Anti-inflammatory foods work as the best traffic controllers and street cleaners, efficiently orchestrating a return to calm and function. They are not a quick-fix trend or a diet in the fad sense; they are the foundations of a sustainable lifestyle that nourishes, heals, and sustains.

Discovering these foods is like unlocking a treasure chest of well-being. They include colorful fruits like cherries and blueberries, hearty leafy greens such as kale and spinach, and robust healthy fats found in avocados and olive oil. It's a cornucopia of choices that tantalise the taste buds while championing your health. Who knew that the humble olive oil drizzled over a fresh salad could be your ally against inflammation, or that sweet, juicy berries could double up as delicious soldiers in your body's defense against oxidative stress and pain?

Amidst our discovery, there are myths to dispel. For years, fats were painted as villains in the nutritional world, but now we understand that healthy fats — those unsaturated ones that solicit a ripple of approval from your heart — are pivotal. They are the prudent mediators, promoting the production of anti-inflammatory eicosanoids, our bodies' own version of peacekeepers.

Lean proteins, too, stand proudly in the anti-inflammatory arsenal. They stride with purpose, repairing and building, ensuring our muscles stay robust and resilient. When we speak of proteins, envision wild-caught salmon dancing in streams, its omega-3 fatty acids a powerful balm to inflammation, or a piece of tender, grilled chicken breast – easy to prepare and packed with potential.

We must not forget the ancient wisdom of spices and herbs, which have long been allies in healing practices around the world. Turmeric, with its golden hue, has been revered for its curcumin content, a compound that scientific studies now laud for its anti-inflammatory prowess. Ginger, too, brings its zesty spark to the table, offering potent anti-inflammatory and antioxidant benefits.

Whole grains and legumes join the chorus, their fibrous structures and nutrient profiles aligning perfectly with the anti-inflammatory melody. They ensure a slow and steady release of energy, keeping blood sugar levels balanced, which is crucial in curbing inflammatory reactions. Aside from their individual merits, what cements these foods' place in our anti-inflammatory journey is their ability to work synergistically. Together, they create a symphony within our bodies that dampens the flames of inflammation, while simultaneously providing rich nutrients that fortify us against future flare-ups.

Embracing these foods means more than just placating physical inflammation; it's about reviving the very essence of wellbeing. Notice that we, too, are like carefully balanced ecosystems. When our internal environment is at peace, it radiates outward, influencing every part of our lives. Our sleep deepens, our energy returns, our minds clear, and our moods lift. It's a holistic transformation, one that ripples outward to touch our families, our work, and our joys.

As we illuminate our plates with bright, anti-inflammatory fare, we light a path back to some of the purest joys of life. The joy found in savoring a meal rich with flavors and benefits, the joy in feeling an energy once believed lost, and the joy in nurturing our loved ones with the same transformative power.

Every journey begins with a single step, or in our case, a single bite. Feeding your body with anti-inflammatory foods isn't just about eating differently; it's about reshaping your life's path towards lasting wellness. It's about standing in the serenity of your kitchen, choosing ingredients with purpose, and embarking on a culinary voyage that charts a course through the tempest of inflammation towards the calm shores of vitality and rejuvenation.

And as your guide, dear reader, nothing brings me greater joy than to be the compass in your hand. Together, let's sail towards a horizon where pain dissipates, energy overflows, and every meal is a chance to nourish not just our bodies, but our very souls.

EMBRACING A NEW LIFESTYLE: MORE THAN JUST FOOD

Embarking on a journey toward better health is akin to setting out on a grand adventure—with all its highs, lows, and transformative experiences. The transition to an anti-inflammatory lifestyle is about more than just substituting ingredients in your pantry or revamping your menu. It is about embracing a holistic approach to well-being, one that encompasses not only the food you eat but also the mindset you adopt and the habits you cultivate.

Picture this diet as a garden: the foods are the seeds, but your lifestyle is the soil. For those seeds to flourish, the ground must be fertile and well-tended. As you read through these pages, I invite you to consider the broader scope of your life, examining how stress management, physical activity, and even the little moments of joy you allow yourself can be a balm to inflammation.

Often, inflammation is branded as an outright villain. However, it's important to recognize that it's a natural response of your immune system, crucial in protecting and healing your body. The goal is to pacify the chronic, unchecked inflammation that overstays its welcome, leading to discomfort and a myriad of health issues. Your choices—the way you unwind after a long day, the sleep you prioritize at night, even the relationships you nurture—these too knead the dough of a nourishing life.

Let's delve into what it truly means to live an anti-inflammatory life. Sure, peppering your favorite dishes with turmeric or sipping on green tea are toe-dips into a vast pool. But how about the way you savor your meals, or the slow stretches you perform upon waking, greeting the day with care? How about the laughter-filled evenings spent with loved ones, or the wind-kissed walks in nature? It's remarkable how these threads intertwine, crafting a tapestry that supports your body's natural balance.

Integral to this transformation is understanding that small, consistent changes accumulate over time. They don't need to be seismic shifts. In fact, the most sustainable alterations are those made incrementally; a gentle steering of the ship rather than a jarring about-face. Give yourself permission to evolve at your own pace. You don't have to leap into a 5 a.m. yoga routine or forage for exotic berries—unless, of course, that brings you joy.

Consider instead how you might integrate mindful practices into your meals. Do you find yourself mindlessly munching in front of the computer? Could you instead set the table, even if dining alone, and play some soft music, chew slowly and savor each bite?

Mindfulness extends beyond the dinner plate. It's in the conscious decision to take the stairs rather than the elevator, to park a little further from the grocery store entrance, or to stand and stretch during one's sedentary office job. It's recognizing stress triggers and countering them, perhaps through guided meditations, journaling, or simply by taking deep, intentional breaths. The foundation of this lifestyle is the food, undoubtedly. But if you envision nourishment merely as a collection of meals, you're only skimming the surface. Nourishment is also the care with which you prepare your food, the gratitude with which you receive it, and the company with which you share it.

When it comes to food, joy and satisfaction shouldn't be casualties of your healthful quest. A common misconception is that by steering toward an anti-inflammatory diet, one must forfeit flavors and culinary pleasures. On the contrary, this pathway opens up a spectrum of tastes, textures, and aromas: think of the zest of fresh herbs, the creamy embrace of avocado, the char and smokiness from a perfectly grilled vegetable. Eating healthfully not only satisfies your body's needs but also satiates your gastronomic desires.

Shifting toward a healthier lifestyle may unearth the need for changes beyond your diet. The environments we inhabit—both at home and work—play significant roles in our overall well-being. Cultivating a space that invites tranquility and creativity can do wonders for one's state of mind, which in turn influences the body's inflammatory responses. This might mean decluttering your space, adding plants to your desk, or ensuring that your bedroom is a sanctuary designed for restful sleep.

Mutual support is invaluable in this journey. Whether it's the camaraderie you find in a cooking class, the shared commitment with a friend to try new anti-inflammatory recipes each week, or the conversations with loved ones about this mutual path toward health—you are not alone.

As we move forward together, remember to cherish the process as much as the outcomes. Celebrate the small victories: the successful preparation of a meal, the newfound vitality, the mornings you wake up with less stiffness in your joints. Be compassionate with yourself on the days when things don't go as planned; they're part of the landscape, too, offering their own lessons and opportunities for growth.

In the forthcoming chapters, I'll guide you through the nuts and bolts of which foods will be your allies in this quest, but always within the larger context that nourishment is all-encompassing. It's about food, yes, but it's also about the life you wrap around that food—the pleasure, the habits, the care. Let's embark on this journey together, savoring each step, each bite, each breath we take towards a more vibrant life.

THE ANTI-INFLAMMATORY DIET: A COMPREHENSIVE GUIDE

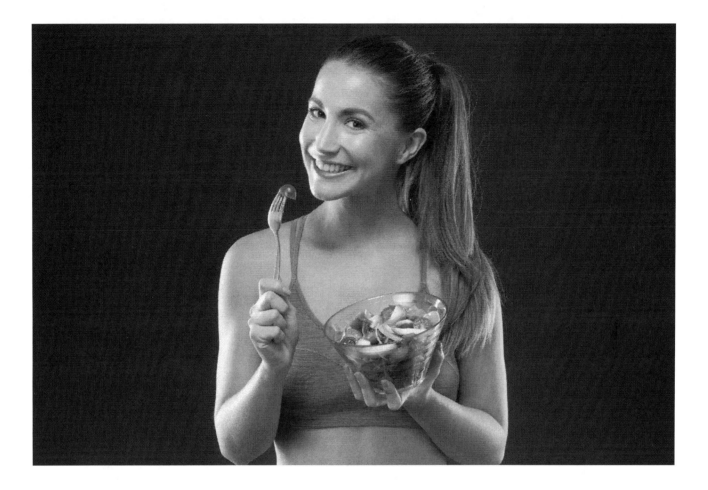

DETAILED OVERVIEW OF THE DIET, INCLUDING ITS BENEFITS AND PRINCIPLES.

Embarking on an anti-inflammatory dietary journey can feel as much like untangling a ball of wool as it does discovering a new way of life. Yet, the simplicity and elegance with which our bodies communicate their gratitude for good nutrition is a symphony worth tuning into. The principles underlying the anti-inflammatory diet are straightforward, yet profound in their capacity to heal and invigorate.

Imagine your body as a finely tuned machine; it thrives on premium fuel—nutrients that dampen inflammation, a biological response akin to fire in the body. Chronic low-grade inflammation is like a smoldering ember that can ignite a host of diseases, from arthritis to heart disease, diabetes to dementia. Yet, with the right culinary toolkit, you can douse these flames and set a course for vibrant health.

The anti-inflammatory diet isn't about loss; it's about love—love for the foods that love us back. It is abundant in plant-based foods, rich in omega-3 fatty acids, and generous with herbs and spices that have been revered since ancient times for their healing properties. It cuts back on processed foods, sugars, and trans fats—those ingredients which tend to fan the flames of inflammation.

Here's a glimpse into the benefits of this healthful paradigm; a diet that doesn't just ward off disease but also promotes an exuberance for life. It eases chronic pain, dials down the risk of developing countless ailments, and supports mental health. Moreover, it paves the way for a robust immune system, adept at fending off infections and more. As inflammation subsides, you might notice an increased pep in your step, a sharper mental clarity, and a connectivity with your body that you hadn't deemed possible.

The tapestry of an anti-inflammatory diet is woven with a few core principles:

Fresh, Whole Foods:

The foundation of this diet is fresh produce. Vibrantly colored fruits and vegetables are not just mere decoration on your plate; they are loaded with antioxidants, vitamins, and minerals. They're the sentinels keeping watch over our well-being.

Balance is Key:

Like a tightrope walker, the anti-inflammatory diet is about balance—specifically, the balance of fats. Not all are foes. Omega-3 fats, found in fish like salmon and seeds such as flax and chia, are champions in reducing inflammation. Conversely, omega-6 fats, while necessary, can promote inflammation when consumed in excess.

Whole Grains and Fiber:

Befriend fiber-rich foods like brown rice, quinoa, and oats, which are slow to digest and steady the rise in blood sugar levels. Not only do whole grains make for an efficient energy source, but they also play a pivotal role in digestive health, which is inextricably linked to our overall inflammatory status.

Power of Protein:

Choosing the right proteins is akin to picking your dance partners; they must be in tune with your body. Lean proteins such as chicken, turkey, and plant-based sources align harmoniously with the goal of reducing inflammation.

The Spice of Life:

Herbs and spices are more than flavor enhancers; they're potent anti-inflammatory agents. Turmeric, ginger, garlic, and cinnamon—these are just a few of the many jewels in nature's treasure chest that are renowned for their anti-inflammatory prowess.

Savoring Healthy Fats:

This diet showers praises on the healthy fats that come from nuts, seeds, and certain oils like olive oil. They aren't merely condiments to cooking, but compounds that carry the torch of inflammation-reduction across every cell in your body.

Hydration for Healing:

Water acts as the body's natural transport system, a vital contributor to reducing inflammation. Herbal teas, too, provide a soothing avenue and are rife with antioxidative properties.

Limit Inflammatory Culprits:

It's no great reveal that certain indulgences poke at inflammation like a stick to a hornet's nest. Sugar, processed foods, and excessive red meat consumption aren't just taxing on the waistline but on our internal ecosystem as well.

The adoption of this diet does not demand a regimented adherence to rigidity. Rather, it embraces flexibility and personalization. Listening to your body is vital; it will guide you to what best soothes your inflammation, what energy levels it sustains, and even the moods it nurtures. It is a diet crafted not just of ingredients but of intuition—a custom blend of what nurtures your unique physiology.

As you journey through these pages, remember that each recipe, each meal plan, is a stepping stone to a fuller, more vibrant life. You're not just cooking; you're concocting remedies, sprinkling healing, and weaving wellness into your everyday existence. There's a certain poetry to food, and in the anti-inflammatory diet, you're both the author and the audience of a transformative narrative of health.

IDENTIFYING AND UNDERSTANDING INFLAMMATORY TRIGGERS IN YOUR DIET

In the realm of health and well-being, the food choices we make are akin to selecting the fabric of our daily lives. Some fabrics are rough and irritative, while others soothe and comfort. Our diet, replete with various ingredients, functions in much the same way—certain foods cause inflammation, akin to that itchy wool sweater, while others are the soft cotton that nurtures our body.

Being mindful of what we eat is paramount because sometimes the culprits triggering inflammation are stealthy, hidden in plain sigh within meals we consider innocuous or even healthy. These inflammatory triggers cause our immune system to go into defense mode, leading to chronic inflammation, which is like a smoldering fire within your body. It's not the overt, acute inflammation you get with a sprained ankle or a bee sting – that kind of inflammation comes and goes and is a natural part of healing. Chronic inflammation, on the other hand, is subtle and persistent, and it has been implicated in a host of health issues, from arthritis to heart disease, diabetes to Alzheimer's.

You might be thinking, "But Isabel, how can I know which foods inflame and which foods soothe?" Let's embark on this journey of discovery together.

Firstly, ultra-processed foods are the modern marauders of tranquility. Laden with artificial additives, preservatives, and high levels of sugar and salt, they can provoke an inflammatory response. Think of processed meats, sugary cereal, and snacks that come packaged with long shelf lives – these can disrupt the harmony in your body.

Refined carbohydrates are like the false friends of the food world—they promise quick energy but lead to spikes in blood sugar and insulin, setting the stage for inflammation. White bread, pastries, and other baked goods made from white flour are the usual suspects here.

Another contentious group is excessive omega-6 fatty acids. These are essential fats, sure, but in today's diets, we often consume them in disproportion to their anti-inflammatory counterparts, omega-3s. The imbalance can promote inflammation. Omega-6s are ubiquitous in many vegetable oils and, by extension, in many foods we prepare with these oils.

Next, trans fats are akin to the body's foes in disguise. Hiding in margarine, fried foods, and many commercially baked goods, they don't just raise the bad LDL cholesterol but also incite inflammatory responses.

Now, while dairy can be a nutritious part of many diets, for some individuals, dairy products—particularly those from cow's milk—can lead to inflammation, especially for those with a sensitivity or intolerance to lactose or casein.

Red meat and processed meats, loved by many for their rich flavor, can also be problematic. These foods not only contain saturated fats but also molecules such as Neu5Gc, which the human body does not naturally produce and can recognize as a foreign threat, potentially resulting in inflammation.

Sugar—oh, how sweet and yet pernicious it is! High intake of added sugars, like those found in sodas, candy, and even seemingly healthy juices, is akin to laying out the red carpet for inflammation.

Lastly, and perhaps surprisingly, certain vegetable and seed oils that are high in omega-6 fatty acids, like sunflower, safflower, and corn oil, can also contribute to the imbalance that leads to inflammation.

Now you may be wondering, "How can I tell if these foods are affecting me?" It's a blend of self-awareness and trial and error. Start by scrutinizing ingredient labels when you shop. Are there any trans fats hiding in your favorite packaged items? Is sugar infiltrating in as an unnecessary reinforcement? Gradually phase out ultra-processed foods, opting instead for whole, unprocessed choices.

It's also about tuning into your body's signals. After consuming certain foods, do you feel sluggish, bloated, or experience a vague sense of discomfort? These may be your body's whispering protests against inflammatory insurgents. Keeping a food diary can help you connect the dots—note down what you eat and how you feel afterward. Over time, patterns may emerge, clues guiding you towards a more anti-inflammatory path.

Some people find that an elimination diet, where you remove common inflammatory foods like gluten, dairy, and sugar for a while and then gradually reintroduce them, can help determine what your body reacts to. But remember, always consult with a healthcare provider before significantly altering your diet, especially if you have health conditions or are on medication.

And what about those moments of longing for the comforting foods that now seem forbidden? Recognize that it is not about creating a list of villainous foods never to be enjoyed again. It is more about striking a balance, learning moderation, and understanding the impact of these foods on your body. It's also about finding joy in the bountiful options still available to you—foods rich in antioxidants, fiber, omega-3 fatty acids, and other nutrients that can help quell the flames of inflammation.

Transitioning to an anti-inflammatory diet isn't about deprivation; it's about transformation. It's a chance to reimagine your palate, explore new flavors, and rediscover the innate wisdom of eating food as nature intends. Consider each meal an opportunity to nourish and heal, a small yet significant step on the journey to better health. Remember, a life free from chronic pain and full of vibrancy is well within reach, and it all starts with the simplest of choices—what you put on your plate today.

SYNERGIZING DIET WITH LIFESTYLE FOR OPTIMAL HEALTH

Embarking on the journey to embrace an anti-inflammatory diet extends far beyond the perimeters of what we pile onto our plates. It is a wholesome dance between the foods we choose and the lives we lead—a symbiotic relationship, where one informs and enriches the other. Nourishing your body is an act of self-care, but to truly observe the benefits, we need to synergize our diet with our lifestyle for optimal health.

Imagine each day as a canvas on which you are the artist. You wield the power to create a vibrant and harmonious masterpiece or a discordant array of strokes. Integrating anti-inflammatory foods into your diet is akin to selecting vivid, life-affirming colors to fill your day. What this synergy entails is a series of intentional choices that align with the nutrition you infuse your body with.

Let's consider our sleeping habits to start. The embrace of restorative sleep is a key ally to an anti-inflammatory diet. When sleep and diet hold hands, the body's repair mechanisms engage more robustly, inflammation quiets down, and you wake up rejuvenated. Aim for seven to nine hours of quality sleep each night, and you may just find that the wholesome foods of your daytime fuel a deeper, more peaceful slumber.

Moving our bodies is like stirring the pot—it mixes and blends our internal landscape, enhancing how we absorb and utilize nutrients. Exercise, even in gentle, regular doses, can dramatically boost your body's anti-inflammatory responses. Marry a brisk thirty-minute walk with a diet abundant in leafy greens and omega-rich fish, and you are orchestrating a bodily symphony of well-being.

But, let's also talk about managing something we all grapple with: stress. Chronic stress can wreak havoc on your body, lighting the fires of inflammation in a continuous, relentless assault. The right diet, brimming with antioxidants, can provide your armor. Pair this with stress-reducing practices like mindfulness, meditation, or even simple breathing exercises, and you are creating a fortress that buffers you from the siege of stress. The tranquility in your mind will reflect in the tranquility of your body.

While diet plays an indispensable role, let's not forget about the liquids that flow through our lives—hydration. Water is the essence of life and the elixir that facilitates our body's anti-inflammatory functions. Make it a habit to sip water throughout the day. Infuse it with anti-inflammatory herbs or a slice of lemon for an added twist of detoxification. Stay hydrated and watch as this simple act magnifies the impact of every fiber-rich vegetable, every antioxidant-packed berry you consume.

In our interconnected lives, the community we build becomes a part of this dietary lifestyle synergy. Sharing meals creates bonds and these bonds can reinforce our commitment to the anti-inflammatory path. Building a community, whether it is a Sunday family dinner ritual or a potluck with friends where everyone brings a dish rich in colorful vegetables and whole grains, fosters support, accountability, and joy in the journey.

Now I know changing habits is no easy feat—it demands courage and an unwavering resolve. But as you align your diet with these life habits, you enter a state of grace where everything flows together, enhancing each other. It's like a beautifully composed symphony where every note is essential—the diet, the sleep, the exercise, the stress management, the hydration, and the community—each one plays its part in creating a state of optimal health and vitality.

As we maneuver through the complexities of life, finding balance can seem as perplexing as a labyrinth. Yet it is the mainstay of your anti-inflammatory journey. It's not just about what you eat, but also when you eat. Regular meal times set your body's rhythm, supporting circadian cycles and ensuring that every organ works in harmony. Early dinners, coupled with an overnight fast, can prove to be an effective tandem in reducing inflammation and supporting gut health.

Yet, with all these lifestyle choices swirling around us, remember the cornerstone of it all—the joy to be found in this journey. Like the aromatic herbs that add zest to your dish, sprinkle elements of joy into your life. Cultivate hobbies, laugh often, connect deeply, and infuse a spirit of gratitude for the nourishment and the life you are creating. It is this zest that transforms the journey from a prescriptive diet to a cherished way of life.

So, dear readers, the art of synergizing diet with lifestyle is much akin to learning a delicate dance. It's about embracing the rhythm, the ebb and flow of everyday choices that lead to a life lived well—a life where chronic pain and inflammation are not uninvited guests, but rather, distant memories. As you close the covers of this chapter, carry with you the knowledge that each step you take on this path is a step towards a veritable symphony of health that your body and soul so richly deserve.

NAVIGATING YOUR PANTRY: WHAT TO KEEP AND WHAT TO DISCARD

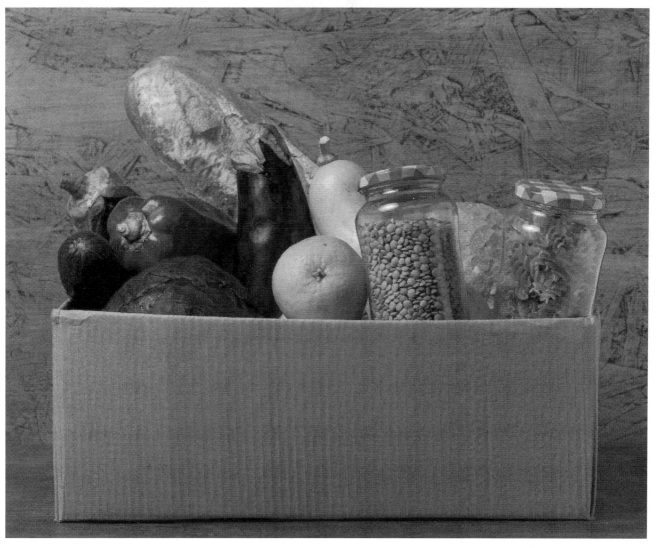

PRACTICAL ADVICE ON ORGANIZING THE KITCHEN WITH ANTI-INFLAMMATORY FOODS AND ELIMINATING HARMFUL ITEMS.

Embarking on a journey of anti-inflammatory eating is like setting sail on a voyage to better health—one where your kitchen is the commanding ship, your pantry the valued cargo, and you, my dear reader, the skilled captain. Your pantry's contents determine much of your diet's success, so let's carefully chart a course through which items to stock and which to drop anchor on and leave behind.

Imagine your pantry as a garden where you'll sow seeds of nourishment; the choices you make now will sprout into your future well-being. To pave the path to vibrant health, you'll want to first create an environment conducive to anti-inflammatory eating. Start by combing through your current provisions. Identify any processed foods with long ingredient lists, as these often include additives and preservatives that incite inflammation. Banish refined sugars and flours, hydrogenated oils, and anything with more numbers than a lottery ticket.

Now, to replenish with bountiful choices that support your health objectives. Consider your pantry like a palette for an artist—stock up on a variety of colors and textures, focusing on whole, unprocessed foods. Let's paint a picture of what that looks like:

Whole Grains:

Swap those refined grains for their whole counterparts. A treasure trove of fiber, these grains are stalwarts in the anti-inflammatory kitchen. Quinoa, brown rice, oats, and barley not only offer versatility in your culinary creations but also help stabilize blood sugar levels, which is essential in reducing inflammation.

Nuts and Seeds:

Almonds, walnuts, chia seeds, and flaxseeds are like little nuggets of anti-inflammatory gold. They're rich in Omega-3 fatty acids, which act as the body's natural anti-inflammatory agents. Sprinkle them into your morning oatmeal or whip up a homemade trail mix for a healthful snack.

Legumes:

Beans and lentils may be humble, but they pack a mighty nutritional punch. Abundant in protein, they are also high in fiber and antioxidants, aiding in the squelching of inflammation. They're versatile, too; work them into soups, salads, or even make them the star of a dish in a hearty bean stew.

Herbs and Spices:

Curcumin in turmeric, allicin in garlic, gingerol in ginger—these are not just culinary agents of flavor but powerful anti-inflammatory substances. Keeping a well-stocked spice rack can transform the ordinary into the extraordinary while bestowing upon your meals their inflammation-fighting prowess.

Healthy Oils:

Swap out those vegetable oils high in Omega-6 fatty acids for bottles brimming with Omega-3 and monounsaturated fats. Extra virgin olive oil and avocado oil not only dress your salads but also bathe your cells in a protective layer against inflammation.

Vinegars and Acidic Elements:

Apple cider vinegar and fresh lemon juice are not only zesty additions to salad dressings but are also believed to have alkalizing effects on the body, creating an environment less hospitable to inflammation.

Canned Goods:

When selecting canned items, like tomatoes or pumpkin, opt for those with no added salt or sugars. Better yet, choose items packed in water or their own juice with BPA-free lining to ensure you're not inadvertently welcoming unwanted chemicals into your wholesome diet.

After filling your pantry with these beneficial foods, commit to being vigilant about expiration dates and proper storage. Maintaining order in your cache will not only keep it fresh and usable but will also serve as a visual reminder of your commitment to health each time you reach for a snack or begin meal prep.

This shift in your pantry is emblematic of a shift in your life—one that may require a period of adjustment, as any significant change does. But remember, each ingredient you choose to include or exclude is a step towards the vibrant health you yearn for—and you're not just revamping a shelf space, you're revolutionizing your diet, one spice jar, one bag of quinoa at a time.

Nevertheless, be gentle with yourself. At times, temptation may beckon you toward old habits, but with a well-stocked arsenal and the wisdom of healthy choices at your fingertips, you're more than equipped to fend off such siren calls. You do not need to be perfect. Small, steady alterations lead to lasting change.

Recognize, too, the economic aspect of overhauling your pantry. It doesn't need to happen overnight, nor should it compromise your wallet's wellbeing. Introduce items gradually, perhaps aligning with the lifecycle of your current supplies. And bear in mind: the cost of anti-inflammatory foods may seem higher at the checkout, but measured against medical expenses and lost days of vibrant living, it's a worthy investment your future self will thank you for.

As we conclude this leg of the journey, look at your renewed pantry with pride. It's a reflection of your commitment to your health and a physical manifestation of your determination to live pain-free, energized, and fully nourished. So here's to you, and the delicious, healing recipes that await you—may your meals be as joyful as they are restorative. Bon voyage and bon appétit!

Stocking Up: Essential Anti-Inflammatory Ingredients

Embarking on an anti-inflammatory journey can feel as thrilling as setting sail on uncharted waters. You are the captain of your ship, and your pantry is the hold where you'll stock the provisions necessary for a successful voyage. To reach a territory free of chronic pain and abundant in health, we must ensure our pantry is filled with the right kind of sustenance.

Essential anti-inflammatory ingredients are the cornerstone of your nutritional treasure chest. These staples not only add flavor and diversity to your meals but also stand as allies in your quest to reduce inflammation and bolster your immune system. Let's embark on the delightful task of stocking up!

Wholesome Oils and Fats

Akin to the oil that keeps a lantern burning bright, healthy fats will be the light guiding you on your path. Extra virgin olive oil reigns supreme with its monounsaturated fats and polyphenols, which are known to ease inflammation. Let's also embrace avocado oil, with its creamy texture and versatility, and coconut oil, a tropical treasure that adds a hint of sweetness and is brilliant for baking. Don't forget the omega-3 rich flaxseed and chia seed oils, which are excellent for drizzling over salads.

Grains and Seeds – The Fibrous Treasures

The hulls of our ship are strengthened with the fibrous might of whole grains such as quinoa, old-fashioned oats, and brown rice. These grains are teeming with fiber, crucial for digestive health. Remember that consistency is key – integrating these into your daily routine will keep the sails of your health billowing.

We also can't overlook seeds - chia, flax, hemp, and pumpkin seeds are veritable nuggets of nutrition. They're packed with anti-inflammatory omega-3 fatty acids and can be sprinkled on breakfast bowls, woven into baking, or just nibbled as a snack.

Fruits and Vegetables – The Rainbow Crew

A diverse crew is vital to a ship's success, much like a variety of fruits and vegetables is to your body. Strive to include every color of the rainbow on your plate. Deep greens of spinach and kale, the vibrant blues and purples of berries and eggplant, and the bold reds of tomatoes and bell peppers; each hue represents a host of different antioxidants and phytonutrients essential for taming inflammation.

Let's not forget the root cellar of our vessel where we store anti-inflammatory stalwarts like beets, sweet potatoes, and turmeric – these earthy gems offer a grounding force in your flavorful creations.

Herbs and Spices – The Flavor Pioneers

Herbs and spices are small but mighty; they are the compass that points our meals in the right direction. Think of fresh ginger and turmeric as your navigators, steering you away from the reefs of inflammation. Include garlic, which sails against the wind of high blood pressure, and cinnamon, which helps regulate your blood sugar. Fresh herbs like basil, parsley, and cilantro add not just a burst of flavor to dishes but also significant health benefits.

Legumes and Nuts – The Protein Deckhands

On this journey, legumes and nuts perform the vital task that young deckhands do aboard a galleon – they work vigorously behind the scenes. Black beans, lentils, chickpeas, and other legumes are high in fiber and plant-based protein; they keep our ship steady and support our muscles and tissues. Nuts like almonds, walnuts, and Brazil nuts provide healthy fats and are a convenient, satisfying snack.

Fish and Lean Meats – The Catch of the Day

Although this part of the pantry might be in your refrigerator or freezer, it's no less important. Fish like wild salmon, mackerel, and sardines are teeming with anti-inflammatory omega-3 fatty acids. When considering meats, opt for pasture-raised chicken or turkey and grass-fed beef. These choices are not only lean but also higher in beneficial omega-3s compared to their conventionally raised counterparts.

Fermented Foods – Probiotic Pirates

Let's not marginalize the beneficial bacteria that should populate our gut – they are the probiotic pirates that protect our treasure. Incorporate fermented foods like sauerkraut, kimchi, and kefir into your diet. They'll help keep your digestive system in shipshape by balancing your gut flora.

As you stock up on these anti-inflammatory ingredients, visualize your meals transforming into colorful, nutritious, and healing feasts. Take delight in the knowledge that you're paving a path to improved health with every bite you take.

In closing, think of your pantry as a treasure map to health. With each of these ingredients, you add a piece to the puzzle that is your optimal diet. While there is no one-size-fits-all approach to curbing inflammation, these staples lay a vibrant foundation upon which to build a lifestyle robust with health, energy, and, dare I say, a newfound zest for the culinary arts.

Bon voyage, dear reader, as you set sail toward the horizon of wellbeing. With your pantry properly provisioned, you're well-equipped to weather the storms of inflammation and embark on a culinary adventure that promises both taste and vitality.

UNDERSTANDING LABELS: MAKING INFORMED CHOICES AT THE GROCERY STORE

In the bustling aisles of your local grocery store, a symphony of labels beckons from every shelf. Each brightly colored package boasts a host of claims — "low-fat," "heart-healthy," "all-natural" — but what do they truly mean? As we journey together to embrace an anti-inflammatory lifestyle, it is essential to become discerning readers of labels, transforming each shopping trip into an informed foray into nutrition. Let's unveil the mystery behind these labels and learn how to make choices that are truly good for our bodies.

Stepping into the grocery store, the first item that may catch your eye is a bag of chips claiming to be "reduced sodium." It's a term that implies health consciousness, but what lurks beneath the surface could be less benign. "Reduced" often means that the sodium content is merely lower than the original product, not that it is low in sodium. Compare these products to others on the shelf or, better yet, to whole foods that naturally contain minimal sodium. Remember, dear reader, that less does not always equate to little.

Equally beguiling are the "low-fat" and "fat-free" labels. While these products may seem ideal for an anti-inflammatory diet, they frequently compensate for the lack of fat with added sugars or artificial sweeteners, which can silently contribute to inflammation. Our bodies require healthy fats — think avocados, nuts, and olive oil — to reduce inflammation and absorb essential, fat-soluble nutrients. So, be wary of these labels, and don't eschew all fats; instead, focus on the quality of the fat.

Turning to another common label, "gluten-free" has become a buzzword, suggestive of health. While vital for those with celiac disease or gluten intolerance, gluten-free itself is not indicative of anti-inflammatory properties. Many gluten-free products are high in processed flours and sugars, which may conflict with our anti-inflammatory goals. Be judicious, my friends; gluten-free is not intrinsically synonymous with healthy.

The allure of "all-natural" is powerful, tugging at our instincts to eat as nature intended. It conjures images of lush fields and bountiful harvests but take heed: "natural" is not a regulated term, and its presence on a package guarantees neither health benefits nor a lack of processed ingredients. Seek transparency and simplicity in ingredients. If the list is long and filled with unpronounceable words, it may be wise to reconsider.

In a similar vein, "organic" label signifies produce and other items cultivated without synthetic pesticides, fertilizers, and other unwelcome additives. While organic is generally a righteous path in our anti-inflammatory quest, I must urge you to weigh the cost and accessibility against your needs and budget. Prioritize organic for items known to be high in pesticide residues, like berries and leafy greens, but don't feel defeated if not everything in your pantry bears the organic seal.

Now, let us address the siren song of "sugar-free." While reducing sugar is a cornerstone of anti-inflammatory eating, the devil is often in the details — or, in this case, the alternative sweeteners. Artificial sweeteners can still elicit an inflammatory response or impact insulin sensitivity. Look instead for natural sweeteners, used sparingly, such as honey or maple syrup, which may offer antioxidant benefits along with their sweetness.

The conundrum of the "multigrain" and "whole grain" labels is one we must also untangle. "Multigrain" merely indicates that a product contains multiple types of grains, not that they are whole or unprocessed. "Whole grain," however, ensures that all parts of the grain are used, providing fiber, vitamins, and minerals vital for our anti-inflammatory journey. Always verify by checking that whole grains are listed as the primary ingredient.

Lastly, "no added hormones" or "antibiotic-free" labels, often found on meats and dairy, promise a product free of these additives. These are valuable for reducing your exposure to substances that could potentially disrupt your body's natural hormone balance or contribute to antibiotic resistance. They align with our anti-inflammatory aims, but be mindful of the broader nutritional profile of the meat or dairy you choose.

Armed with this knowledge, you are now prepared to navigate the labels that line the grocery store shelves. Embrace the process as part of your culinary adventure. With practice, discerning the truly healthful options will become second nature, and the foods you bring into your kitchen will be ones chosen with confidence and care.

Together, as we continue our voyage toward vibrant health, revel in the empowerment of making informed choices. And rest assured, while the grocery store's labyrinth of labels may seem daunting, every step you take is one toward nourishment, vitality, and a pain-free existence. Treasure the journey, for it is surely as significant as the destination.

BREAKFASTS RECIPES TO KICKSTART YOUR DAY

Wake up to a morning filled with the promise of health and vitality with these anti-inflammatory breakfast recipes designed to nourish and energize your body. These carefully curated dishes combine the wisdom of nutritional science with the art of cooking to provide you with delicious options that fit into your busy lifestyle. Each recipe features wholesome ingredients that work in harmony to reduce inflammation and kickstart your day with flavor and nutrients.

SAVORY SPINACH AND SWEET POTATO HASH

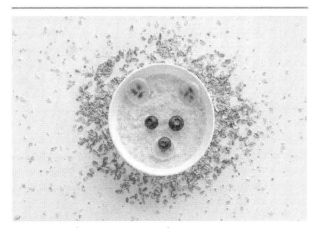

PT: 15 min - **CT:** 25 min
MODE: Stovetop - **SERVS:** 2
INGREDIENTS: 1 large sweet potato, cubed

- 2 Tbls extra virgin olive oil
- 1 tsp smoked paprika
- 1/2 tsp ground cumin
- 1/4 tsp ground turmeric
- 1/2 red onion, diced
- 1 garlic clove, minced
- 2 C. fresh spinach
- 4 free-range eggs
- Sea salt to taste
- Freshly ground black pepper to taste

DIRECTIONS: Preheat a large skillet over medium heat with olive oil

- Add sweet potatoes, paprika, cumin, and turmeric, sauté until they start to soften

- Add red onion and garlic, continue to cook until onion is translucent

- Add spinach and cook until wilted

- Create four wells in the hash and crack an egg into each well

- Cover with a lid and cook until eggs are set

- Season with salt and pepper

TIPS: Top with your favorite hot sauce for added flavor

- Serve with avocado slices for an extra dose of healthy fats

NUTRITIONAL VALUES: Calories: 320 - Fat: 18g - Carbs: 27g - Protein: 14g - Sugar: 6g

CHIA SEED AND COCONUT MILK PORRIDGE

PT: 5 min - **CT:** 15 min
MODE: Stovetop - **SERVS:** 2
INGREDIENTS: 1/4 C. chia seeds

- 1 C. coconut milk
- 1/4 C. flaxseed meal
- 1 Tbls unsweetened almond butter
- 1 tsp pure maple syrup
- 1/2 tsp ground cinnamon
- 1/4 tsp pure vanilla extract
- Pinch of sea salt
- Assorted berries for topping

DIRECTIONS: Combine chia seeds, coconut milk, flaxseed meal, almond butter, maple syrup, cinnamon, vanilla extract, and salt in a pot over medium heat

- Stir constantly until the mixture thickens to a porridge-like consistency

- Remove from heat and let it sit for a couple of minutes

- Serve in bowls with a generous helping of berries on top

TIPS: Stir in a scoop of your favorite plant-based protein powder for an extra morning boost

- Sweeten naturally with fresh fruits or a drizzle of raw honey instead of maple syrup

NUTRITIONAL VALUES: Calories: 255 - Fat: 19g - Carbs: 16g - Protein: 8g - Sugar: 3g

ANTI-INFLAMMATORY BLUEBERRY SMOOTHIE BOWL

PT: 10 min - **CT:** 0 min
MODE: Blender - **SERVS:** 1
INGREDIENTS: 1/2 C. frozen blueberries

- 1/2 banana
- 1 C. spinach
- 1 Tbls ground flaxseed
- 1 Tbls pumpkin seeds
- 1 tsp grated ginger
- 3/4 C. unsweetened almond milk
- Unsweetened coconut flakes for topping
- Hemp seeds for topping

DIRECTIONS: Blend blueberries, banana, spinach, flaxseed, pumpkin seeds, ginger, and almond milk until smooth

- Pour into a bowl and top with coconut flakes and hemp seeds

TIPS: Experiment with different toppings such as cacao nibs or sliced almonds

- For a thinner consistency, add more almond milk

NUTRITIONAL VALUES: Calories: 287 - Fat: 9g - Carbs: 45g - Protein: 10g - Sugar: 19g

ANTI-INFLAMMATORY TURMERIC SCRAMBLE

PT: 5 min - **CT:** 10 min
MODE: Stovetop - **SERVS:** 1
INGREDIENTS: 3 free-range eggs

- 1 Tbls coconut oil
- 1/4 tsp ground turmeric
- 1/4 tsp garlic powder
- 1/4 C. diced red bell pepper
- 1/4 C. diced zucchini
- 2 Tbls nutritional yeast
- Fresh cilantro for garnish
- Sea salt to taste
- Black pepper to taste

DIRECTIONS: In a bowl, whisk eggs with turmeric and garlic powder

- Heat coconut oil in a skillet on medium heat

- Sauté bell pepper and zucchini until tender

- Pour in the egg mixture and cook, occasionally stirring, until eggs are scrambled and fully cooked

- Stir in nutritional yeast

- Serve with fresh cilantro, and season with salt and pepper

TIPS: Add a side of fermented vegetables like kimchi for digestive health benefits

- Serve on a bed of baby spinach to increase your vegetable intake

NUTRITIONAL VALUES: Calories: 330 - Fat: 25g - Carbs: 6g - Protein: 21g - Sugar: 3g

Mushroom and Kale Frittata Muffins

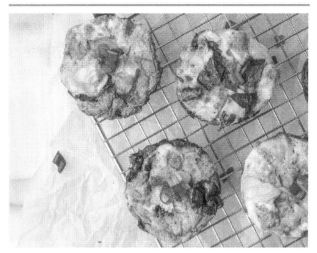

PT: 15 min - **CT:** 25 min
MODE: Oven - **SERVS:** 6
INGREDIENTS: 1 C. kale, chopped

- 3/4 C. cremini mushrooms, sliced

- 6 free-range eggs

- 1/4 C. almond milk

- 1/2 tsp dried oregano

- 1/4 C. grated dairy-free cheese

- 1/2 Tbls extra virgin olive oil

- Sea salt to taste

- Black pepper to taste

DIRECTIONS: Preheat oven to 350°F (175°C)

- Sauté kale and mushrooms in olive oil until soft

- In a bowl, whisk eggs, almond milk, oregano, salt, and pepper

- Stir in sautéed veggies and cheese

- Pour into greased muffin cups

- Bake for 20-25 min or until set

TIPS: For a touch of heat, add a pinch of red pepper flakes to the egg mixture

- Leftovers can be stored in the fridge for a quick breakfast on the go

NUTRITIONAL VALUES: Calories: 130 - Fat: 9g - Carbs: 3g - Protein: 9g - Sugar: 1g

Buckwheat and Zucchini Pancakes

PT: 10 min - **CT:** 20 min
MODE: Griddle - **SERVS:** 4
INGREDIENTS: 1 C. buckwheat flour

- 1 C. grated zucchini

- 1 1/4 C. almond milk

- 1 free-range egg

- 1 Tbls extra virgin olive oil

- 1 tsp baking powder

- 1/2 tsp sea salt

- 1/4 tsp ground nutmeg

- Coconut oil for cooking

DIRECTIONS: Combine buckwheat flour, zucchini, almond milk, egg, olive oil, baking powder, salt, and nutmeg in a bowl and mix until smooth batter forms

- Heat a griddle with coconut oil

- Pour batter to form pancakes, cook until bubbles form on the surface, then flip

- Cook until the other side is golden brown

TIPS: Top with a dollop of unsweetened applesauce for a naturally sweet complement

- To maintain their inherent crispness, serve these pancakes fresh off the griddle

NUTRITIONAL VALUES: Calories: 220 - Fat: 10g - Carbs: 27g - Protein: 7g - Sugar: 4g

Ginger-Infused Oatmeal with Poached Pears

PT: 10 min - **CT:** 30 min
MODE: Stovetop - **SERVS:** 2
INGREDIENTS: 1/2 C. rolled oats

- 1 C. water

- 1 C. almond milk

- 1 ripe pear, halved and cored

- 1 tsp freshly grated ginger

- 1 cinnamon stick

- 1 Tbls chia seeds

- Pinch of sea salt

- Walnuts for topping

- Drizzle of honey for topping

DIRECTIONS: Combine water, almond milk, and a cinnamon stick in a pot and bring to a boil

- Add oats, grated ginger, and salt, reduce heat to a simmer, stir occasionally

- Simmer until oats are tender

- Poach pear halves in the oatmeal until softened

- Serve oatmeal with pear halves on top, sprinkled with chia seeds and walnuts, and finished with a drizzle of honey

TIPS: Customize with your choice of nut butter swirled into the oatmeal

- Substitute honey with maple syrup for a different flavor profile

NUTRITIONAL VALUES: Calories: 275 - Fat: 8g - Carbs: 45g - Protein: 9g - Sugar: 16g

AVOCADO TOAST WITH TOMATO AND PUMPKIN SEEDS

PT: 5 min - **CT:** 5 min

MODE: Toaster - **SERVS:** 1

INGREDIENTS: 2 slices gluten-free bread

- 1 ripe avocado

- 1/2 small tomato, sliced

- 1 Tbls pumpkin seeds

- 1 Tbls extra virgin olive oil

- 1/2 tsp lemon juice

- 1/4 tsp crushed red pepper flakes

- Sea salt to taste

- Black pepper to taste

DIRECTIONS: Toast gluten-free bread to desired crispness

- In a bowl, mash avocado with lemon juice, red pepper flakes, salt, and pepper

- Spread mashed avocado evenly on toast

- Top with tomato slices and sprinkle with pumpkin seeds and a drizzle of olive oil

TIPS: Squeeze additional lemon juice on top to enhance flavor and preserve the vibrant green color of the avocado

- For an extra kick, add a sprinkle of smoked paprika

NUTRITIONAL VALUES: Calories: 300 - Fat: 22g - Carbs: 24g - Protein: 7g - Sugar: 3g

SAVORY TURMERIC OATMEAL

PT: 10 min. - **CT:** 20 min.

MODE: Stovetop - **SERVS:** 2

INGREDIENTS: 1 C. steel-cut oats

- 1 tsp turmeric powder

- 1/4 tsp black pepper

- 1 Tbls extra virgin olive oil

- 2 C. low-sodium vegetable broth

- 1 C. water

- 1/2 tsp sea salt

- 1/4 C. pumpkin seeds, toasted

- 1/2 C. cherry tomatoes, halved

- 1/4 C. fresh cilantro, chopped

DIRECTIONS: Combine oats, turmeric, pepper, and olive oil in a saucepan over medium heat and toast the oats slightly

- Add the vegetable broth and water, bring to a boil, then simmer, covered, for 20 min.

- Remove from heat and let stand for 2 min.

- Divide between bowls and top with pumpkin seeds, tomatoes, and cilantro

TIPS: Try a dollop of plain Greek yogurt for added creaminess and protein

- Black pepper enhances turmeric absorption, amplifying its anti-inflammatory properties

NUTRITIONAL VALUES: Calories: 315 - Fat: 9g - Carbs: 48g - Protein: 12g - Sugar: 1g

ANTI-INFLAMMATORY SHAKSHUKA

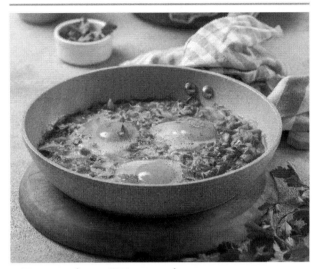

PT: 10 min. - **CT:** 30 min.
MODE: Stovetop - **SERVS:** 4
INGREDIENTS: 2 Tbls avocado oil

- 1 onion, finely chopped
- 2 garlic cloves, minced
- 1 red bell pepper, sliced
- 1 C. tomatoes, diced
- 1 tsp cumin
- 1 tsp smoked paprika
- 4 large eggs
- Sea salt to taste
- Fresh cilantro for garnish

DIRECTIONS: Heat oil in a large skillet, add onion, garlic, and bell pepper and sauté until softened

- Add tomatoes, cumin, and paprika, simmer for 20 min. to blend flavors

- Create wells in the sauce and crack the eggs into each

- Cover and cook until eggs are done to your liking

- Season with salt and garnish with cilantro

TIPS: Serve with gluten-free toast or a side of sauteed greens

- Add a pinch of cayenne for an extra anti-inflammatory kick

NUTRITIONAL VALUES: Calories: 220 - Fat: 14g - Carbs: 12g - Protein: 12g - Sugar: 5g

CHIA AND HEMP SEED PARFAIT

PT: 15 min. - **CT:** 0 min.
MODE: No Cooking - **SERVS:** 2
INGREDIENTS: 1 C. unsweetened almond milk

- 3 Tbls chia seeds
- 2 Tbls hemp seeds
- 1/2 tsp vanilla extract
- 2 Tbls pure maple syrup
- 1 C. mixed berries
- 1/4 C. gluten-free granola

DIRECTIONS: Mix almond milk, chia seeds, hemp seeds, vanilla extract, and maple syrup in a bowl and let it sit for 15 min. until it reaches a pudding-like consistency

- Layer chia pudding with berries and granola in parfait glasses

TIPS: For extra anti-inflammatory benefit, sprinkle with cinnamon

- Prepare the night before for a quick, grab-and-go breakfast

NUTRITIONAL VALUES: Calories: 280 - Fat: 14g - Carbs: 32g - Protein: 8g - Sugar: 12g

WARM GINGER-PEAR BREAKFAST SALAD

PT: 15 min. - **CT:** 5 min.
MODE: Stovetop - **SERVS:** 4
INGREDIENTS: 4 ripe pears, cubed

- 1 Tbls fresh ginger, minced
- 1/2 tsp ground cinnamon
- 1 Tbls coconut oil
- 1/4 C. dried cranberries
- 1/4 C. walnuts, chopped
- 2 tsp honey

DIRECTIONS: Heat coconut oil in a skillet over medium heat

- Add ginger and cinnamon, cooking until fragrant, about 1 min.
- Add pears and cook until tender, 5 min.
- Remove from heat, mix in cranberries, walnuts, and drizzle with honey
- Serve warm

TIPS: Serve over plain yogurt for added protein and probiotics

- Walnuts can be replaced with pecans for a different flavor profile

NUTRITIONAL VALUES: Calories: 180
- Fat: 7g - Carbs: 29g - Protein: 2g - Sugar: 20g

GOLDEN MILK STEEL-CUT OAT RISOTTO

PT: 5 min. - **CT:** 35 min.
MODE: Stovetop - **SERVS:** 2
INGREDIENTS: 1/2 C. steel-cut oats

- 1 can light coconut milk
- 1 C. water
- 2 Tbls honey
- 1 tsp ground turmeric
- 1/2 tsp ground cinnamon
- 1/4 tsp ground ginger
- 1 pinch ground black pepper
- 1 Tbls coconut oil
- 1 Tbls flax seeds

DIRECTIONS: Combine coconut milk, water, honey, turmeric, cinnamon, ginger, and pepper in a saucepan and bring to a gentle simmer

- Add oats and cook, stirring occasionally, for 35 min. until creamy
- Stir in coconut oil and flax seeds before serving

TIPS: Top with your favorite nuts for added texture and omega-3 fatty acids

- Stir occasionally to prevent sticking and achieve a creamy risotto-like texture

NUTRITIONAL VALUES: Calories: 300
- Fat: 11g - Carbs: 44g - Protein: 6g - Sugar: 9g

MISO-INFUSED SCRAMBLED EGGS

PT: 5 min. - **CT:** 10 min.
MODE: Stovetop - **SERVS:** 2
INGREDIENTS: 4 large eggs

- 1 Tbls miso paste
- 1 Tbls water
- 1 Tbls grass-fed butter
- 1 green onion, finely sliced
- 1/2 tsp toasted sesame seeds

DIRECTIONS: In a bowl, whisk together eggs, miso paste, and water until well combined

- Melt butter in a nonstick pan over medium heat
- Pour in the egg mixture and cook, stirring gently, until softly set
- Top with green onion and sesame seeds

TIPS: Serve with a side of fermented vegetables for a gut-health boost

- Using a nonstick pan helps to achieve the perfect scramble texture without adding excess fat

NUTRITIONAL VALUES: Calories: 230 - Fat: 17g - Carbs: 2g - Protein: 16g - Sugar: 1g

AVOCADO AND WHITE BEAN TOAST

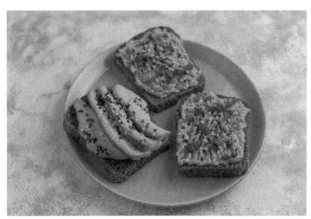

PT: 10 min. - **CT:** 2 min.
MODE: Toaster & Stovetop - **SERVS:** 2
INGREDIENTS: 1 ripe avocado
- 1/2 C. white beans, cooked
- 1 Tbls lemon juice
- Sea salt to taste
- Red pepper flakes to taste
- 2 slices gluten-free bread, toasted
- 1/2 C. arugula
- 1 tsp extra virgin olive oil

DIRECTIONS: Mash avocado and white beans together with lemon juice, salt, and red pepper flakes
- Spread mixture on toasted bread
- Top with arugula and a drizzle of olive oil

TIPS: Enhance the flavors with a sprinkle of nutritional yeast
- Use fresh, high-quality extra virgin olive oil for a flavorful finish

NUTRITIONAL VALUES: Calories: 310 - Fat: 14g - Carbs: 38g - Protein: 10g - Sugar: 3g

CINNAMON QUINOA BREAKFAST BOWL

PT: 15 min. - **CT:** 25 min.
MODE: Stovetop - **SERVS:** 2
INGREDIENTS: 1 C. quinoa, rinsed
- 2 C. almond milk
- 1/2 tsp ground cinnamon
- 1 Tbls almond butter
- 2 Tbls raisins
- 1 apple, diced
- 1 Tbls chia seeds
- 1 tsp pure maple syrup

DIRECTIONS: Combine quinoa, almond milk, and cinnamon in a pot and bring to a boil
- Reduce heat to low and simmer, covered, for 25 min. until quinoa is cooked and liquid is absorbed
- Stir in almond butter, raisins, and apple
- Top each bowl with chia seeds and a drizzle of maple syrup

TIPS: Customize with your favorite seasonal fruits or nuts
- Sweeten naturally with a touch of maple syrup or honey if preferred

NUTRITIONAL VALUES: Calories: 320 - Fat: 9g - Carbs: 53g - Protein: 9g - Sugar: 12g

SHAKSHUKA WITH LEAFY GREENS

PT: 10 min. - **CT:** 20 min.
MODE: Stovetop - **SERVS:** 4
INGREDIENTS: 1 Tbls extra virgin olive oil

- 1 small onion, finely chopped
- 2 garlic cloves, minced
- 1 bell pepper, diced
- 1 tsp cumin
- ½ tsp smoked paprika
- ¼ tsp coriander
- A pinch of cayenne pepper
- 1 can (14 oz.) diced tomatoes
- 4 large free-range eggs
- 2 C. baby spinach
- ¼ C. crumbled feta cheese
- Fresh cilantro for garnish
- Salt and pepper to taste

DIRECTIONS: Heat oil in a large skillet and sauté onion, garlic, and bell pepper until softened

- Add cumin, paprika, coriander, cayenne, and season with salt and pepper, cooking for another minute until aromatic
- Pour in diced tomatoes and simmer for about 10 minutes until thickened
- Stir in baby spinach until wilted
- With a spoon, make wells in the sauce and crack eggs into each well
- Cover and cook until eggs are set to your liking
- Sprinkle with feta and cilantro before serving

TIPS: Serve with gluten-free toast or warm flatbread to keep it anti-inflammatory

- Adjust the level of cayenne to regulate spiciness as needed
- For added richness, a dollop of coconut yogurt can be added atop each serving

NUTRITIONAL VALUES: Calories: 220 - Fat: 12g - Carbs: 15g - Protein: 14g - Sugar: 8g

MILLET & APPLE BREAKFAST BAKE

PT: 15 min. - **CT:** 45 min.
MODE: Oven - **SERVS:** 6
INGREDIENTS: 2 C. millet, rinsed

- 4 C. unsweetened almond milk
- 2 large apples, peeled and chopped
- 1/3 C. dried cranberries
- 2 Tbls coconut sugar
- ½ tsp nutmeg
- ½ tsp ground ginger
- 1 tsp pure vanilla extract
- ¼ C. crushed walnuts
- Preheat oven to 375°F (190°C)

DIRECTIONS: In a casserole dish, combine millet, almond milk, apples, cranberries, coconut sugar, nutmeg, and ginger

- Stir in vanilla extract and mix thoroughly
- Cover with aluminum foil and bake for 35 minutes
- Remove the foil, sprinkle with crushed walnuts, and bake uncovered for another 10-15 minutes until the top is golden and millet is cooked through

TIPS: Incorporate a tablespoon of flaxseed meal for an omega-3 boost

- Serve with a drizzle of almond butter for extra creaminess and flavor
- Leftovers can be stored in the refrigerator for an effortless breakfast the next day

NUTRITIONAL VALUES: Calories: 260 - Fat: 5g - Carbs: 48g - Protein: 6g - Sugar: 15g

SPIRULINA & COCONUT PORRIDGE

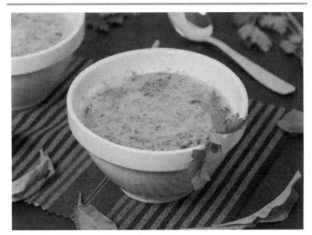

PT: 5 min. - **CT:** 10 min.
MODE: Stovetop - **SERVS:** 2
INGREDIENTS: 1 C. rolled oats

- 2 C. almond milk
- 1 Tbls spirulina powder
- 1 Tbls chia seeds
- 1 ripe banana, mashed
- 1 Tbls raw honey
- ½ tsp cinnamon
- A pinch of sea salt
- Toasted coconut flakes for garnish
- Fresh berries for serving

DIRECTIONS: Combine almond milk, oats, and sea salt in a pot and bring to a simmer over medium heat

- Stir in spirulina, chia seeds, and mashed banana, cooking until oats are tender and porridge is creamy

- Remove from heat and stir in cinnamon and raw honey

- Serve garnished with toasted coconut flakes and fresh berries

TIPS: Opt for organic spirulina for purity and enhanced health benefits

- Honey can be substituted with maple syrup for a vegan option

- Add a scoop of your favorite protein powder for an extra boost

NUTRITIONAL VALUES: Calories: 295 - Fat: 4g - Carbs: 54g - Protein: 9g - Sugar: 12g

GOLDEN TURMERIC YOGURT BOWL

PT: 5 min. - **CT:** 0 min.
MODE: No Cooking - **SERVS:** 1
INGREDIENTS: 1 C. Greek yogurt

- 1 Tbls turmeric
- 1 Tbls raw honey
- 2 Tbls pumpkin seeds
- 1 Tbls goji berries
- ½ ripe mango, diced
- 1 Tbls ground flaxseed
- 1 tsp ground cinnamon

DIRECTIONS: Mix Greek yogurt with turmeric, honey, and cinnamon until well combined

- Top with pumpkin seeds, goji berries, diced mango, and a sprinkle of ground flaxseed

TIPS: Select a probiotic-rich yogurt to support gut health

- Customize with your favorite seasonal fruits or nuts

- If you prefer plant-based yogurt, ensure it is fortified with calcium and vitamin D for added benefits

NUTRITIONAL VALUES: Calories: 310 - Fat: 10g - Carbs: 36g - Protein: 18g - Sugar: 28g

SAVORY OATMEAL WITH AVOCADO AND POACHED EGG

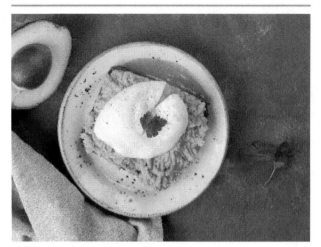

PT: 10 min. - **CT:** 15 min.
MODE: Stovetop - **SERVS:** 1
INGREDIENTS: ⅓ C. steel-cut oats

- ¾ C. vegetable broth

- 1 free-range egg

- ½ an avocado, sliced

- 1 Tbls nutritional yeast

- 1 tsp apple cider vinegar

- 1 Tbls olive oil

- Salt and pepper to taste

- 1 Tbls pumpkin seeds

- Chopped chives for garnish

DIRECTIONS: Cook steel-cut oats in vegetable broth according to package instructions until creamy

- In a separate pot, bring water to a gentle simmer and add apple cider vinegar

- Crack egg into a small dish and gently slide into simmering water for poaching

- Cook for 4 minutes for a soft yolk

- Top cooked oatmeal with avocado slices, poached egg, and a sprinkle of nutritional yeast, pumpkin seeds, chives, salt, and pepper

TIPS: Enhance the savory flavor with a few drops of tamari

- A sprinkle of hemp seeds can be added for extra protein and omega-3 fatty acids

- Poaching the egg in broth infuses additional flavor

NUTRITIONAL VALUES: Calories: 345
- Fat: 20g - Carbs: 27g - Protein: 16g - Sugar: 1g

CHIA AND RASPBERRY BREAKFAST PUDDING

PT: 10 min. - **CT:** 2 hr. chill time
MODE: Refrigerator - **SERVS:** 2
INGREDIENTS: ¼ C. chia seeds

- 1 C. coconut milk

- 1 C. raspberries

- 1 Tbls maple syrup

- ½ tsp almond extract

- 1 Tbls slivered almonds

- 1 tsp lemon zest

DIRECTIONS: Combine chia seeds with coconut milk, half of the raspberries, maple syrup, and almond extract, stirring well

- Chill in the refrigerator for at least 2 hours, or overnight, until thickened

- Serve topped with remaining raspberries, slivered almonds, and lemon zest

TIPS: The pudding can be sweetened further if needed, using a touch of stevia or additional maple syrup

- For a refreshing twist, mint leaves can be added

- Chia pudding can be layered with additional fruits and nuts for a parfait-like experience

NUTRITIONAL VALUES: Calories: 280
- Fat: 19g - Carbs: 24g - Protein: 6g - Sugar: 8g

SALADS AND VEGETABLES RECIPES

Within these pages lies a cornucopia of salads and vegetable dishes, each crafted to enliven your plate and soothe your body with their anti-inflammatory bounty. As we unveil these recipes, imbued with vibrant colors and diverse textures, we celebrate the fortifying power of nature's gifts. These culinary creations are not merely food; they are your allies in a quest for a life less inflamed, a dance of flavors and nutrients designed to nourish and delight.

RAINBOW CHARD AND POMEGRANATE SALAD

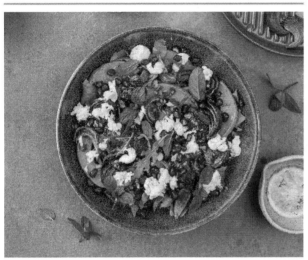

PT: 15 min - **CT:** 0 min
MODE: No Cooking - **SERVS:** 4
INGREDIENTS: 1 bunch rainbow chard, stems removed and leaves thinly sliced

- 1 C. pomegranate arils

- ½ C. walnuts, toasted and roughly chopped

- 3 Tbls extra virgin olive oil

- 1 Tbls apple cider vinegar

- 1 tsp Dijon mustard

- 1 garlic clove, minced

- Himalayan pink salt to taste

- Freshly ground black pepper to taste

DIRECTIONS: Whisk together extra virgin olive oil, apple cider vinegar, Dijon mustard, minced garlic, salt, and pepper to create the dressing

- In a large bowl, toss together the rainbow chard, pomegranate arils, and walnuts
- Drizzle the dressing over the salad and toss gently to coat evenly

TIPS: Massage the chard leaves with a bit of the dressing to tenderize them before adding the other ingredients

- Toast the walnuts to enhance their nutty flavor and add a delightful crunch

NUTRITIONAL VALUES: Calories: 210 - Fat: 16g - Carbs: 16g - Protein: 4g - Sugar: 7g

JICAMA AND ORANGE CITRUS BURST SALAD

PT: 20 min - **CT:** 0 min
MODE: No Cooking - **SERVS:** 4
INGREDIENTS: 1 medium jicama, julienned

- 3 navel oranges, peeled and cut into segments

- ⅓ C. red bell pepper, finely diced

- ¼ C. fresh cilantro, chopped

- 1 Tbls lime juice

- 1 Tbls raw honey

- Himalayan pink salt to taste

- Freshly ground black pepper to taste

DIRECTIONS: In a serving bowl, combine julienned jicama, orange segments, red bell pepper, and chopped cilantro

- Whisk together lime juice and raw honey for the dressing, season with salt and pepper

- Pour dressing over the salad ingredients and toss gently until well mixed

TIPS: Jicama adds not only a crisp texture but also acts as a prebiotic, supporting gut health

- Chill the salad before serving to allow flavors to meld

NUTRITIONAL VALUES: Calories: 130 - Fat: 0.5g - Carbs: 31g - Protein: 2g - Sugar: 22g

BEETROOT CARPACCIO WITH ARUGULA AND FETA

PT: 15 min - **CT:** 0 min
MODE: No Cooking - **SERVS:** 4
INGREDIENTS: 3 medium beets, cooked and thinly sliced

- 2 C. arugula

- ⅓ C. feta cheese, crumbled

- ¼ C. walnuts, crushed

- 2 Tbls balsamic reduction

- 1 Tbls extra virgin olive oil

- Freshly ground black pepper to taste

- Himalayan pink salt to taste

DIRECTIONS: Arrange beet slices on a plate, overlapping slightly

- Scatter arugula over the beets

- Sprinkle crumbled feta and crushed walnuts on top

- Drizzle balsamic reduction and extra virgin olive oil over the salad

- Season with salt and pepper to taste

TIPS: Serve immediately after drizzling with balsamic to maintain the crispness of the arugula

- The earthy sweetness of beetroot pairs delightfully with the tanginess of balsamic reduction

NUTRITIONAL VALUES: Calories: 124 - Fat: 7g - Carbs: 12g - Protein: 4g - Sugar: 9g

KOHLRABI SLAW WITH GINGER LIME DRESSING

PT: 15 min. - **CT:** 0 min.
MODE: No Cooking - **SERVS:** 4
INGREDIENTS: 1 large kohlrabi, peeled and grated

- 2 carrots, grated

- 1/4 red cabbage, finely shredded

- 2 scallions, thinly sliced

- For Ginger Lime Dressing: 2 Tbls lime juice

- 1 Tbls grated fresh ginger

- 1/4 C. extra virgin olive oil

- 1 Tbls apple cider vinegar

- 1 tsp honey

- Salt and pepper to taste

DIRECTIONS: In a large bowl, mix together kohlrabi, carrots, red cabbage, and scallions

- Whisk together the dressing ingredients and pour over the slaw, tossing well to coat

TIPS: Let the slaw sit for 10 min. before serving to allow flavors to meld

- Top with toasted sesame seeds for added texture and nuttiness

NUTRITIONAL VALUES: Calories: 180 - Fat: 14g - Carbs: 12g - Protein: 2g - Sugar: 7g

WARM SPINACH AND MUSHROOM SAUTE

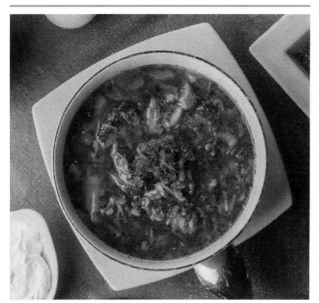

PT: 10 min - **CT:** 15 min
MODE: Sauteing - **SERVS:** 4
INGREDIENTS: 4 C. fresh spinach

- 1 C. shiitake mushrooms, sliced

- 1 Tbls extra virgin olive oil

- 2 Tbls shallots, minced

- 1 garlic clove, minced

- 2 Tbls pine nuts, toasted

- 1 Tbls balsamic vinegar

- Salt to taste

- Freshly ground black pepper to taste

DIRECTIONS: Heat extra virgin olive oil in a large pan over medium heat

- Saute shallots and garlic until translucent, about 3 min

- Add shiitake mushrooms and cook until tender, about 5 min

- Add spinach and saute until just wilted, about 2 min

- Stir in toasted pine nuts and balsamic vinegar

- Season with salt and pepper to taste

TIPS: Sauteing spinach preserves its nutritional profile better than boiling

- Add a sprinkle of nutritional yeast for a cheese-like flavor and extra nutrients

NUTRITIONAL VALUES: Calories: 95 - Fat: 7g - Carbs: 7g - Protein: 3g - Sugar: 2g

KALE AND AVOCADO MASSAGED SALAD

PT: 20 min - **CT:** 0 min
MODE: No Cooking - **SERVS:** 2
INGREDIENTS: 2 C. kale, destemmed and chopped

- 1 ripe avocado, pitted and cut into cubes

- 1 Tbls lemon juice

- 1 Tbls extra virgin olive oil

- 1 tsp raw honey

- ¼ tsp sea salt

- ⅛ tsp crushed red pepper flakes

- ¼ C. red onion, thinly sliced

- 2 Tbls hemp seeds

DIRECTIONS: In a large bowl, add kale, lemon juice, extra virgin olive oil, honey, sea salt, and red pepper flakes

- Massage the kale with hands until it starts to soften and wilt, about 5 min

- Gently fold in avocado cubes and red onion slices

- Top with hemp seeds before serving

TIPS: Massaging kale tenderizes the leaves, making them more palatable and easier to digest

- The creamy avocado acts as a natural dressing, enhancing the salad's richness

NUTRITIONAL VALUES: Calories: 290 - Fat: 22g - Carbs: 21g - Protein: 7g - Sugar: 5g

MIZUNA AND ROASTED ROOT VEGETABLE SALAD

PT: 15 min. - **CT:** 30 min.
MODE: Roasting - **SERVS:** 4
INGREDIENTS: 2 medium beets, peeled and cubed

- 1 large sweet potato, peeled and cubed

- 1 Tbls extra virgin olive oil

- 1 pinch sea salt

- 1 bunch mizuna greens, roughly chopped

- 1/2 red onion, thinly sliced

- 1/4 C. walnuts, toasted and chopped

- For Dressing: 3 Tbls balsamic vinegar

- 1 Tbls Dijon mustard

- 1 clove garlic, minced

- 1/2 C. extra virgin olive oil

- Salt and pepper to taste

DIRECTIONS: Preheat oven to 425°F (220°C)

- Toss beets and sweet potatoes with 1 Tbls olive oil and sea salt, spread on a baking sheet, roast until tender and caramelized, about 30 min.

- Whisk together dressing ingredients, adjust seasoning with salt and pepper

- Combine roasted vegetables, mizuna, red onion in a large bowl, drizzle with dressing, and toss until well coated

- Garnish with toasted walnuts

TIPS: Add goat cheese crumbles for a creamy twist

- Serve warm or at room temperature to best enjoy the flavors

NUTRITIONAL VALUES: Calories: 295 - Fat: 20g - Carbs: 24g - Protein: 4g - Sugar: 9g

CHARRED BROCCOLINI WITH LEMON HERB VINAIGRETTE

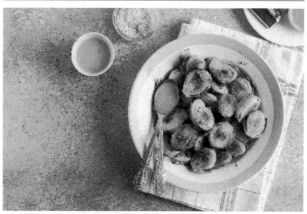

PT: 5 min - **CT:** 10 min
MODE: Grilling - **SERVS:** 4
INGREDIENTS: 1 lb. broccolini, ends trimmed

- 1 Tbls grapeseed oil

- Salt to taste

- Freshly ground black pepper to taste

- Zest of 1 lemon

- 1 Tbls lemon juice

- 1 garlic clove, minced

- 2 Tbls extra virgin olive oil

- 1 Tbls fresh parsley, finely chopped

- 1 Tbls fresh basil, finely chopped

DIRECTIONS: Preheat grill to medium-high heat

- Toss broccolini in grapeseed oil, salt, and pepper

- Grill broccolini until charred in spots, about 10 min, turning occasionally

- For the vinaigrette, combine lemon zest, lemon juice, minced garlic, extra virgin olive oil, chopped parsley, and basil

- Drizzle over the grilled broccolini

TIPS: Charring the broccolini brings out a nutty flavor that complements the bright vinaigrette

- Serve alongside grilled poultry or fish for a meal rich in lean protein and greens

NUTRITIONAL VALUES: Calories: 110 - Fat: 7g - Carbs: 10g - Protein: 3g - Sugar: 2g

SPICY ROASTED CAULIFLOWER WITH TAHINI

PT: 10 min - **CT:** 25 min
MODE: Roasting - **SERVS:** 4
INGREDIENTS: 1 large head of cauliflower, cut into florets

- 2 Tbls avocado oil
- 1 tsp smoked paprika
- ½ tsp turmeric
- ¼ tsp cayenne pepper
- Salt to taste
- 3 Tbls tahini
- 1 Tbls lemon juice
- 1 garlic clove, minced
- 1 Tbls warm water
- Sesame seeds for garnish

DIRECTIONS: Preheat oven to 400°F (200°C)

- Toss cauliflower florets with avocado oil, smoked paprika, turmeric, cayenne pepper, and salt
- Spread evenly on a baking sheet and roast until golden, about 25 min
- For the sauce, whisk tahini, lemon juice, minced garlic, and warm water until smooth
- Drizzle tahini sauce over roasted cauliflower and garnish with sesame seeds

TIPS: For a smokier taste, roast the cauliflower florets until they start to char slightly

- Serve as a delightful side dish or incorporate into a grain bowl for a hearty meal

NUTRITIONAL VALUES: Calories: 145 - Fat: 9g - Carbs: 15g - Protein: 5g - Sugar: 4g

SHAVED BRUSSELS SPROUT AND MANCHEGO SALAD

PT: 15 min - **CT:** 0 min
MODE: No Cooking - **SERVS:** 4
INGREDIENTS: 1 lb. Brussels sprouts, trimmed

- 1 apple, cored and thinly sliced
- ⅓ C. almonds, toasted and roughly chopped
- 3 oz. Manchego cheese, shaved
- 2 Tbls apple cider vinegar
- 4 Tbls extra virgin olive oil
- 1 Tbls Dijon mustard
- 1 tsp raw honey
- Salt to taste
- Freshly ground black pepper to taste

DIRECTIONS: Slice Brussels sprouts very thinly using a mandoline or sharp knife

- Combine apple slices, toasted almonds, and shaved Manchego cheese with the Brussels sprouts in a large bowl
- Whisk together apple cider vinegar, extra virgin olive oil, Dijon mustard, raw honey, salt, and pepper to create the dressing
- Toss the salad with the dressing until evenly coated

TIPS: Almonds add a satisfying crunch and a dose of healthy fats

- Use a vegetable peeler to shave Manchego cheese into thin ribbons

NUTRITIONAL VALUES: Calories: 250 - Fat: 19g - Carbs: 16g - Protein: 9g - Sugar: 7g

Jicama and Watercress Salad with Citrus Vinaigrette

PT: 20 min. - **CT:** 0 min.
MODE: No Cooking - **SERVS:** 2
INGREDIENTS: 1 large jicama, julienned
- 1 bunch watercress, stems removed
- 1 orange, supremed
- 1/2 fennel bulb, thinly sliced
- For Citrus Vinaigrette: 2 Tbls fresh orange juice
- 1 Tbls fresh lime juice
- 1 tsp raw honey
- 1/4 C. extra virgin olive oil
- Salt and pepper to taste

DIRECTIONS: Combine jicama, watercress, orange segments, and fennel in a salad bowl
- Whisk citrus vinaigrette ingredients in a small bowl
- Pour the vinaigrette over the salad and toss gently to coat

TIPS: Serve immediately to preserve the crunch of the jicama
- If watercress is too peppery, substitute with baby spinach

NUTRITIONAL VALUES: Calories: 245 - Fat: 14g - Carbs: 30g - Protein: 3g - Sugar: 14g

Charred Broccolini with Tahini Sauce

PT: 10 min. - **CT:** 10 min.
MODE: Sautéing - **SERVS:** 4
INGREDIENTS: 1 lb. broccolini, ends trimmed
- 1 Tbls avocado oil
- 2 cloves garlic, minced
- 1 pinch chili flakes
- Salt to taste
- For Tahini Sauce: 1/4 C. tahini
- 1 Tbls lemon juice
- 1 Tbls apple cider vinegar
- 1/2 tsp tamari
- 1/4 C. warm water, adjust as needed
- 1 clove garlic, minced
- Salt to taste

DIRECTIONS: Heat avocado oil in a large skillet over medium-high heat
- Add broccolini, garlic, chili flakes, and salt, sauté until broccolini is charred but still vibrant, about 10 min.
- Whisk together tahini sauce ingredients until smooth, adding more water if needed for desired consistency
- Drizzle tahini sauce over charred broccolini before serving

TIPS: For an extra crunch, sprinkle with sesame seeds
- Tahini sauce can be made ahead and stored in the fridge

NUTRITIONAL VALUES: Calories: 165 - Fat: 11g - Carbs: 14g - Protein: 5g - Sugar: 3g

Roasted Beetroot and Arugula Symphony

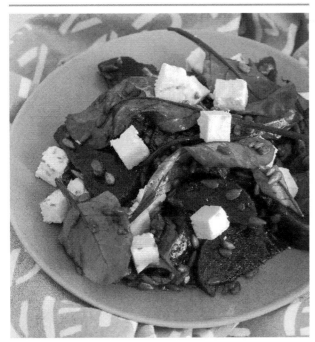

PT: 15 min - **CT:** 25 min
MODE: Roasting - **SERVS:** 4
INGREDIENTS: 3 medium beetroots, peeled and cubed

- 2 C. fresh arugula
- 1/4 C. walnuts, toasted and chopped
- 1/4 C. crumbled feta cheese
- 2 Tbls extra-virgin olive oil
- 1 Tbls balsamic glaze
- 1/2 tsp fresh thyme leaves
- Salt and black pepper to taste

DIRECTIONS: Preheat oven to 400°F (200°C)

- Toss beetroot cubes with 1 Tbls olive oil, salt, and pepper
- Spread on a baking sheet and roast until tender and caramelized
- Let cool slightly
- In a bowl, combine roasted beetroot, arugula, walnuts, and feta cheese
- Drizzle with remaining olive oil and balsamic glaze
- Garnish with thyme before serving

TIPS: Add orange segments for a citrusy twist

- Walnuts can be swapped with toasted pecans for a different nutty profile

NUTRITIONAL VALUES: Calories: 180 - Fat: 14g - Carbs: 10g - Protein: 4g - Sugar: 7g

Spicy Kale and Quinoa Power Bowl

PT: 20 min - **CT:** 15 min
MODE: Boiling - **SERVS:** 2
INGREDIENTS: 1 C. quinoa, rinsed

- 2 C. water
- 1 bunch kale, stems removed and leaves chopped
- 1 ripe avocado, sliced
- 1/2 C. cherry tomatoes, halved
- 1/4 C. red onion, thinly sliced
- 1 Tbls apple cider vinegar
- 2 Tbls extra-virgin olive oil
- 1/2 tsp chili flakes
- Salt and black pepper to taste

DIRECTIONS: In a saucepan, bring quinoa and water to boil

- Reduce heat to simmer, cover, and cook until quinoa is fluffy
- Steam kale until just wilted
- In a large bowl, mix quinoa, steamed kale, avocado slices, cherry tomatoes, and red onion
- Whisk together olive oil, apple cider vinegar, chili flakes, salt, and pepper to make dressing
- Toss salad with dressing until evenly coated

TIPS: Serve with a squeeze of fresh lime juice for extra zest

- A sprinkle of hemp seeds will boost the protein content

NUTRITIONAL VALUES: Calories: 310 - Fat: 14g - Carbs: 40g - Protein: 8g - Sugar: 3g

CARAMELIZED FENNEL AND CITRUS CRUNCH

PT: 10 min - **CT:** 20 min
MODE: Sautéing - **SERVS:** 4
INGREDIENTS: 2 medium fennel bulbs, sliced thin

- 2 Tbls coconut oil
- 1 C. orange segments
- 1/2 C. pomegranate seeds
- 1/2 tsp crushed fennel seeds
- 1 Tbls fresh lemon juice
- 1 Tbls raw honey
- Salt and black pepper to taste

DIRECTIONS: Heat coconut oil in a pan over medium heat

- Add fennel slices and sauté until golden and caramelized
- Lower heat, add crushed fennel seeds, and stir for a minute
- Remove from heat and let cool
- Whisk together lemon juice, honey, salt, and pepper to make dressing
- In a serving bowl, combine caramelized fennel, orange segments, and pomegranate seeds
- Toss with dressing to serve

TIPS: To enhance the fennel's sweetness, add a drizzle of balsamic reduction

- Pair with grilled chicken from Chapter 7 for a complete meal

NUTRITIONAL VALUES: Calories: 165 - Fat: 7g - Carbs: 25g - Protein: 2g - Sugar: 20g

FIERY GINGER-TURMERIC CAULIFLOWER RICE

PT: 10 min - **CT:** 5 min
MODE: Sautéing - **SERVS:** 3
INGREDIENTS: 1 head cauliflower, riced

- 1 Tbls coconut oil
- 1 Tbls fresh ginger, minced
- 1 tsp turmeric powder
- 1/4 C. green onions, sliced
- 1/4 tsp cayenne pepper
- Salt to taste

DIRECTIONS: Heat coconut oil in a large skillet over medium heat

- Add ginger and sauté until fragrant
- Stir in turmeric and cayenne pepper quickly to avoid burning
- Add cauliflower rice and sauté for 5 minutes, until tender
- Remove from heat, toss in green onions and serve

TIPS: Garnish with fresh cilantro for an herbaceous lift

- A squeeze of fresh lime adds a refreshing tang

NUTRITIONAL VALUES: Calories: 80 - Fat: 3.5g - Carbs: 10g - Protein: 3g - Sugar: 4g

Shaved Brussels Sprouts with Warm Bacon Vinaigrette

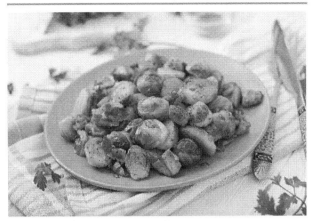

PT: 15 min - **CT:** 10 min
MODE: Sautéing - **SERVS:** 4
INGREDIENTS: 1 lb. Brussels sprouts, trimmed and thinly sliced

- 4 strips sugar-free bacon, diced
- 1 Tbls apple cider vinegar
- 1 tsp Dijon mustard
- 1 Tbls raw honey
- 1/4 C. olive oil
- Salt and freshly ground black pepper to taste

DIRECTIONS: Cook bacon in a pan until crispy

- Remove bacon and set aside, reserving fat in the pan
- Add apple cider vinegar, Dijon mustard, and honey to the pan, whisking to combine
- Slowly whisk in olive oil to emulsify vinaigrette
- Season with salt and pepper
- In a large bowl, toss Brussels sprouts with warm vinaigrette and crispy bacon

TIPS: This salad can double as a warm side dish

- For a vegetarian option, omit bacon and use smoked almonds instead

NUTRITIONAL VALUES: Calories: 240 - Fat: 18g - Carbs: 16g - Protein: 6g - Sugar: 7g

Rainbow Radish and Edamame Salad with Ume Plum Dressing

PT: 15 min - **CT:** 0 min
MODE: No Cooking - **SERVS:** 4
INGREDIENTS: 1 C. radishes, various colors, thinly sliced

- 1 C. shelled edamame, cooked and cooled
- 1/2 C. cucumber, julienned
- 1/4 C. shredded carrots
- 1 Tbls sesame oil
- 2 tsp ume plum vinegar
- 1 tsp raw honey
- Sesame seeds for garnish

DIRECTIONS: In a bowl, combine sliced radishes, edamame, cucumber, and carrots

- In a small bowl, whisk together sesame oil, ume plum vinegar, and honey for dressing
- Drizzle dressing over the salad and toss gently
- Garnish with sesame seeds

TIPS: Experiment by adding seaweed for a marine twist

- Substitute ume plum vinegar with rice vinegar if necessary, adjusting sweetness to taste

NUTRITIONAL VALUES: Calories: 130 - Fat: 6g - Carbs: 13g - Protein: 7g - Sugar: 5g

Chilled Zucchini Ribbon Salad with Lemon-Herb Dressing

PT: 20 min - **CT:** 0 min
MODE: No Cooking - **SERVS:** 2
INGREDIENTS: 2 medium zucchini, cut into ribbons with a vegetable peeler

- 1/4 C. fresh basil leaves, torn
- 2 Tbls fresh lemon juice
- 1/4 C. extra-virgin olive oil
- 1 clove garlic, minced
- 1 Tbls fresh parsley, chopped
- Salt and freshly ground black pepper to taste

DIRECTIONS: Use a vegetable peeler to create thin zucchini ribbons

- In a bowl, whisk together lemon juice, olive oil, garlic, parsley, salt, and pepper to make the lemon-herb dressing

- Toss zucchini ribbons and basil with dressing just before serving

TIPS: Serving chilled enhances the salad's refreshing quality

- Add pine nuts for a toasty crunch

NUTRITIONAL VALUES: Calories: 190 - Fat: 15g - Carbs: 12g - Protein: 2g - Sugar: 7g

CHARRED EGGPLANT WITH POMEGRANATE AND TAHINI DRIZZLE

PT: 15 min - **CT:** 10 min
MODE: Grilling - **SERVS:** 4
INGREDIENTS: 2 large eggplants, halved lengthwise

- 1/4 C. tahini
- 2 Tbls fresh lemon juice
- 1 clove garlic, minced
- 2 Tbls pomegranate seeds
- 1 Tbls fresh mint leaves, chopped
- Salt and black pepper to taste
- Olive oil for grilling

DIRECTIONS: Preheat grill to medium-high heat

- Brush eggplant halves with olive oil and season with salt and pepper

- Grill eggplant, flesh side down, until charred and tender

- Whisk together tahini, lemon juice, and minced garlic to make dressing

- Drizzle dressing over grilled eggplant, garnish with pomegranate seeds and mint

TIPS: Grill lemon halves alongside the eggplant for an extra pop of smoky citrus flavor to add to the dressing

- The tahini dressing can be prepared ahead for convenience

NUTRITIONAL VALUES: Calories: 180 - Fat: 14g - Carbs: 15g - Protein: 3g - Sugar: 9g

HEART-HEALTHY FISH AND SEAFOOD RECIPES

Embark on a heart-healthy voyage with Chapter 6, where the bounty of the sea takes center stage. These eight recipes celebrate the ocean's finest offerings, designed with the anti-inflammatory diet in mind. From the robust flavors of the Mediterranean to the delicate subtleties of Asian-inspired dishes, each creation is not only a delight to the palate but also a steadfast ally to your health. Rejuvenate your body with meals teeming with omega-3s, lean proteins, and a wealth of essential nutrients, all while savoring the rich tapestry of tastes that seafood can provide.

CITRUS-INFUSED SALMON CARPACCIO

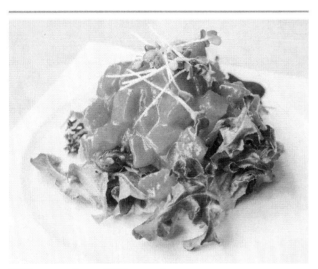

PT: 15 min. - **CT:** 0 min.
MODE: No Cooking - **SERVS:** 4
INGREDIENTS: 1 lb. fresh salmon, skinless

- 1 Tbls extra virgin olive oil
- 2 Tbls fresh orange juice
- 1 Tbls fresh lemon juice
- 1 Tbls capers
- ¼ tsp pink Himalayan salt
- 1/8 tsp cracked black pepper
- ¼ C. fresh dill, chopped
- Zest from one orange

DIRECTIONS: Slice salmon into thin pieces

- Whisk together olive oil, orange juice, lemon juice, salt, and pepper
- Drizzle the mixture over salmon slices
- Garnish with dill, orange zest, and capers

TIPS: Serve immediately for the freshest flavor

- Pair with a crisp, dry white wine for an enhanced dining experience

NUTRITIONAL VALUES: Calories: 191 - Fat: 9g - Carbs: 2g - Protein: 23g - Sugar: 1g

MONKFISH PICCATA WITH CAPERS AND ARTICHOKES

PT: 10 min. - **CT:** 20 min.
MODE: Sautéing - **SERVS:** 4
INGREDIENTS: 1 ½ lb. monkfish fillets

- 2 Tbls almond flour
- ½ tsp paprika
- ¼ C. avocado oil
- 1 Tbls minced garlic
- 1 C. chicken broth, low sodium
- 2 Tbls lemon juice
- ¼ C. capers
- 1 C. artichoke hearts, quartered
- 1 Tbls fresh parsley, chopped
- Salt and pepper to taste

DIRECTIONS: Dust monkfish fillets with almond flour and paprika

- Heat avocado oil over medium, then sauté garlic until golden
- Cook monkfish in oil 4 min. each side, set aside

- Add broth, lemon juice to pan, cook 5 min.

- Stir in capers, artichokes, parsley

- Return monkfish to pan, coat with sauce

TIPS: Pair with steamed asparagus for a complete meal

- Use chicken broth to deglaze the pan and incorporate the fond

NUTRITIONAL VALUES: Calories: 243 - Fat: 10g - Carbs: 6g - Protein: 34g - Sugar: 1g

THAI-STYLE MUSSELS WITH LEMONGRASS BROTH

PT: 15 min. - **CT:** 10 min.
MODE: Steaming - **SERVS:** 4
INGREDIENTS: 2 lb. mussels, cleaned

- 1 can lite coconut milk

- 1 stalk lemongrass, minced

- 1 Tbls ginger, grated

- 2 cloves garlic, minced

- 1 Tbls fish sauce

- 1 Tbls lime juice

- 1 tsp raw honey

- ¼ C. cilantro, roughly chopped

- 1 Tbls coconut oil

- 1 fresh chili, sliced

- Salt to taste

DIRECTIONS: Heat coconut oil in a pot on medium heat

- Sauté lemongrass, ginger, and garlic until aromatic

- Pour in coconut milk, fish sauce, lime juice, and honey, bring to a low boil

- Add mussels, cover and steam until opened, about 8 min.

- Garnish with cilantro and chili

TIPS: Discard any mussels that do not open

- Serve with a side of cauliflower rice for a low-carb option

NUTRITIONAL VALUES: Calories: 295 - Fat: 14g - Carbs: 12g - Protein: 28g - Sugar: 3g

GRILLED SCALLOPS WITH POMEGRANATE SALSA

PT: 10 min. - **CT:** 6 min.
MODE: Grilling - **SERVS:** 4
INGREDIENTS: 12 large sea scallops

- ¼ C. pomegranate seeds

- 1 small avocado, diced

- ¼ C. red onion, finely chopped

- 1 Tbls jalapeño, minced

- 1 Tbls lime juice

- ½ tsp ground cumin

- 1 Tbls cilantro, chopped

- 1 Tbls olive oil

- Salt and pepper to taste

DIRECTIONS: Preheat grill to medium-high (about 400°F/204°C)

- Season scallops with salt, pepper, and brush with oil

- Grill scallops for 3 min. each side until opaque

- Combine pomegranate, avocado, onion, jalapeño, lime juice, cumin, cilantro for salsa

- Top scallops with salsa

TIPS: Avoid moving scallops too much on grill for a good sear

- Pat scallops dry before grilling to ensure proper browning

NUTRITIONAL VALUES: Calories: 197 - Fat: 9g - Carbs: 14g - Protein: 17g - Sugar: 4g

Halibut en Papillote with Julienned Vegetables

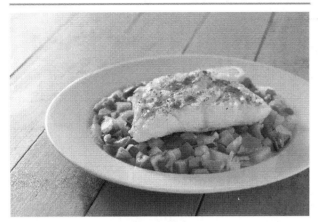

PT: 20 min. - **CT:** 15 min.
MODE: Baking - **SERVS:** 4
INGREDIENTS: 4 halibut fillets, 6 oz. each
  - 1 zucchini, julienned
  - 1 carrot, julienned
  - 1 yellow bell pepper, julienned
  - 2 Tbls dry white wine
  - 4 tsp olive oil
  - 1 Tbls fresh thyme leaves
  - Salt and pepper to taste
  - Parchment paper for wrapping
DIRECTIONS: Preheat oven to 375°F (190°C)
  - Place each fillet on a piece of parchment paper
  - Divide vegetables among the parcels
  - Drizzle each with white wine and olive oil
  - Sprinkle with thyme, salt, and pepper
  - Fold paper over fish, seal edges to form a packet
  - Bake for 15 min.
TIPS: To check if done, fish should flake easily with a fork
  - Let packets sit for a minute before opening to avoid steam burns

NUTRITIONAL VALUES: Calories: 225 - Fat: 7g - Carbs: 6g - Protein: 34g - Sugar: 3g

Pistachio-Crusted Barramundi with Citrus Aioli

PT: 10 min. - **CT:** 12 min.
MODE: Baking - **SERVS:** 4
INGREDIENTS: 4 barramundi fillets, skin on
  - ½ C. pistachios, crushed
  - 1 Tbls dijon mustard
  - 2 Tbls almond flour
  - 1 egg, beaten
  - ½ C. Greek yogurt
  - 1 Tbls orange juice
  - 1 tsp lemon zest
  - Salt and pepper to taste
  - 1 Tbls avocado oil
DIRECTIONS: Preheat oven to 400°F (204°C)
  - Season fish with salt, pepper
  - Spread mustard on fillets, dip in egg, then coat with pistachio and almond flour mix
  - Place on baking sheet with avocado oil
  - Bake for 12 min.
  - Mix Greek yogurt with orange juice, lemon zest for aioli
  - Serve aioli over cooked barramundi
TIPS: Make sure pistachios are crushed finely to stick to fillets
  - Aioli can be prepared ahead and stored in the fridge
NUTRITIONAL VALUES: Calories: 310 - Fat: 15g - Carbs: 9g - Protein: 36g - Sugar: 2g

Grilled Swordfish with Mango Salsa

PT: 20 min. - **CT:** 10 min.

MODE: Grilling - **SERVS:** 4

INGREDIENTS: 4 swordfish steaks, 1 inch thick

- 2 mangos, diced
- ¼ C. red bell pepper, diced
- 1 Tbls fresh mint, chopped
- 1 lime, juiced
- 2 Tbls EVOO
- Sea salt to taste
- Ground black pepper to taste

DIRECTIONS: Season swordfish with salt and pepper

- Grill each side for 5 min. or until cooked through
- Combine mango, red pepper, mint, lime juice, and EVOO to make salsa
- Serve salsa on top of swordfish

TIPS: To avoid overcooking, use high heat and ensure the grill is well-oiled

- Mango salsa can also complement chicken or pork

NUTRITIONAL VALUES: Calories: 330
- Fat: 16g - Carbs: 15g - Protein: 34g - Sugar: 11g

CAJUN BLACKENED COD WITH MANGO AVOCADO SALSA

PT: 15 min. - **CT:** 10 min.

MODE: Pan Frying - **SERVS:** 4

INGREDIENTS: 4 cod fillets, 6 oz. each

- 2 Tbls Cajun seasoning
- 1 mango, diced
- 1 avocado, diced
- ½ red onion, finely chopped
- 1 Tbls lime juice
- 1 Tbls cilantro, chopped
- 1 Tbls coconut oil
- Salt to taste

DIRECTIONS: Season cod fillets with Cajun seasoning and salt

- Heat coconut oil in a skillet over medium-high
- Cook cod for 5 min. on each side until cooked through
- Combine mango, avocado, onion, lime juice, cilantro for salsa
- Serve salsa over blackened cod

TIPS: Do not overcrowd the pan to ensure even cooking and a good crust

- Use ripe but firm mango and avocado for the salsa

NUTRITIONAL VALUES: Calories: 232
- Fat: 9g - Carbs: 13g - Protein: 26g - Sugar: 7g

SCALLOP AGUACHILE WITH CUCUMBER

PT: 15 min. - **CT:** 0 min.

MODE: Chilling - **SERVS:** 4

INGREDIENTS: 12 large sea scallops, thinly sliced

- 1 cucumber, peeled and thinly sliced
- 1 C. fresh lemon juice

- 2 serrano chilies, seeded and sliced

- ¼ C. red onion, thinly sliced

- 2 Tbls EVOO

- Sea salt to taste

- 1 tsp black sesame seeds for garnish

DIRECTIONS: Arrange scallops and cucumber in a shallow dish

- Whisk together lemon juice, EVOO, chilies, and onions, and pour over scallops

- Chill for 15 min. to allow flavors to blend

- Garnish with black sesame seeds and sea salt before serving

TIPS: To keep the delicate texture of the scallops, do not marinate for too long

- Black sesame seeds add a nutty flavor and a visual contrast

NUTRITIONAL VALUES: Calories: 150 - Fat: 7g - Carbs: 8g - Protein: 14g - Sugar: 2g

MISO-MARINATED BLACK COD

PT: 3 hr. - **CT:** 10 min.
MODE: Broiling - **SERVS:** 2
INGREDIENTS: 2 black cod fillets (6 oz. each)

- 1/4 C. white miso

- 2 Tbls mirin

- 2 Tbls sake

- 1 Tbls soy sauce

- 1 Tbls sugar

- 1 tsp grated ginger

- Green onions, sliced for garnish

DIRECTIONS: Combine miso, mirin, sake, soy sauce, sugar, and ginger

- Coat cod evenly with marinade and refrigerate for 3 hr.

- Preheat broiler

- Broil cod until flaky and slightly caramelized, about 10 min.

TIPS: Serve with steamed bok choy and garnish with green onions

- Glaze can be used on other fish varieties

NUTRITIONAL VALUES: Calories: 290 - Fat: 5g - Carbs: 12g - Protein: 42g - Sugar: 7g

CITRUS-INFUSED GRILLED OCTOPUS

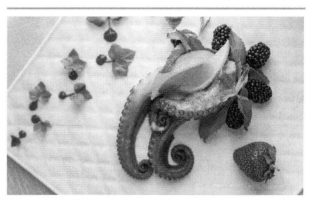

PT: 20 min. - **CT:** 45 min.
MODE: Grilling - **SERVS:** 4
INGREDIENTS: 1 lb. octopus, cleaned

- 2 Tbls extra virgin olive oil

- 1 orange, zested and juiced

- 1 lemon, zested and juiced

- 2 cloves garlic, minced

- 1 tsp smoked paprika

- 1 tsp dried oregano

- Sea salt to taste

- Freshly ground black pepper to taste

DIRECTIONS: Marinate the octopus in citrus juices, zests, and seasonings for 15 min.

- Preheat grill to medium-high heat

- Grill octopus until charred and tender, about 45 min., turning occasionally

TIPS: Serve with a drizzle of olive oil and a sprinkle of fresh parsley

- Pair with a side of quinoa for a complete meal

NUTRITIONAL VALUES: Calories: 175 - Fat: 5g - Carbs: 8g - Protein: 25g - Sugar: 2g

CHILI-LIME SHRIMP WITH ZOODLES

PT: 15 min. - **CT:** 10 min.
MODE: Sautéing - **SERVS:** 4
INGREDIENTS: 1 lb. shrimp, peeled and deveined

- 2 Tbls olive oil
- 1 Tbls chili powder
- Juice of 2 limes
- 4 medium zucchinis, spiralized
- 2 cloves garlic, minced
- Sea salt to taste
- Freshly ground black pepper to taste
- Fresh cilantro, chopped for garnish

DIRECTIONS: Toss shrimp with half the olive oil, chili powder, lime juice, salt, and pepper

- Heat remaining oil in a pan
- Sauté garlic until fragrant
- Add shrimp and cook until opaque
- Toss with spiralized zucchini until warmed through

TIPS: Top with fresh cilantro and additional lime wedges

- Zoodles can be substituted with spaghetti squash for variety

NUTRITIONAL VALUES: Calories: 170 - Fat: 8g - Carbs: 7g - Protein: 20g - Sugar: 5g

CAJUN-SPICED CATFISH WITH COLLARD GREENS

PT: 10 min. - **CT:** 20 min.
MODE: Pan-frying - **SERVS:** 4
INGREDIENTS: 4 catfish fillets (6 oz. each)

- 1 Tbls Cajun spice blend
- 2 Tbls avocado oil
- 1 lb. collard greens, ribs removed and leaves thinly sliced
- 1/2 C. vegetable broth
- 1 Tbls apple cider vinegar
- 2 cloves garlic, minced
- Salt and pepper to taste

DIRECTIONS: Season catfish with Cajun spice

- Heat 1 Tbls oil in a skillet and cook catfish until golden, about 5 min. per side
- Remove and set aside
- In the same skillet, add remaining oil, collard greens, broth, vinegar, and garlic
- Cook until greens are tender

TIPS: Serve collard greens as a bed for the catfish

- The Cajun spice blend can be made at home for a fresher flavor

NUTRITIONAL VALUES: Calories: 215 - Fat: 9g - Carbs: 6g - Protein: 28g - Sugar: 1g

HERB-CRUSTED HADDOCK EN PAPILLOTE

PT: 15 min. - **CT:** 20 min.
MODE: Baking - **SERVS:** 2
INGREDIENTS: 2 haddock fillets (6 oz. each)

- 1 Tbls fresh dill, chopped
- 1 Tbls fresh parsley, chopped
- 2 tsp fresh thyme leaves
- 1 Tbls olive oil
- Salt and pepper to taste
- Parchment paper for wrapping

DIRECTIONS: Preheat oven to 400°F (204°C)

- Mix herbs, olive oil, salt, and pepper
- Coat fish with herb mixture
- Wrap each fillet in parchment paper
- Bake for 20 min. or until fish flakes easily

TIPS: Unwrapping the packet at the table makes for an aromatic presentation

- Pair with roasted asparagus

NUTRITIONAL VALUES: Calories: 190 - Fat: 6g - Carbs: 1g - Protein: 32g - Sugar: 0g

SEARED SCALLOPS WITH POMEGRANATE BEURRE BLANC

PT: 10 min. - **CT:** 15 min.
MODE: Searing - **SERVS:** 4
INGREDIENTS: 12 large sea scallops

- 2 Tbls clarified butter
- 1 shallot, finely diced
- 1/2 C. pomegranate juice
- 1/4 C. white wine
- 1 Tbls heavy cream
- 4 Tbls unsalted butter, cubed
- Salt and pepper to taste
- Fresh pomegranate seeds for garnish

DIRECTIONS: Season scallops with salt and pepper

- Heat clarified butter in a pan
- Sear scallops, about 2 min. per side
- For beurre blanc, soften shallot, add pomegranate juice and wine
- Reduce by half, stir in cream
- Off heat, whisk in butter gradually

TIPS: Garnish with pomegranate seeds

- Beurre blanc can be prepared ahead and gently reheated

NUTRITIONAL VALUES: Calories: 310 - Fat: 18g - Carbs: 10g - Protein: 24g - Sugar: 6g

HARISSA-RUBBED SWORDFISH STEAKS

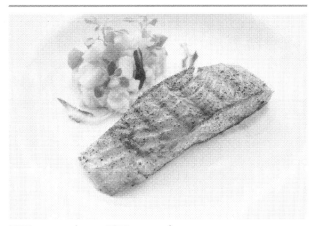

PT: 25 min. - **CT:** 15 min.
MODE: Grilling - **SERVS:** 4
INGREDIENTS: 4 swordfish steaks (6 oz. each)

- 2 Tbls harissa paste
- 1 Tbls olive oil
- Juice of 1 lemon
- 1 tsp ground cumin
- 1 tsp smoked paprika
- Salt and pepper to taste
- Lemon wedges for serving

DIRECTIONS: Combine harissa, olive oil, lemon juice, cumin, and paprika

- Rub mixture over swordfish and let stand for 20 min.
- Preheat grill to medium heat
- Grill swordfish until cooked through, about 6-7 min. per side

TIPS: Brush with extra harissa paste if desired

- Serve with lemon wedges and a side of couscous

NUTRITIONAL VALUES: Calories: 280 - Fat: 10g - Carbs: 2g - Protein: 45g - Sugar: 0g

CHERMOULA-BASTED HALIBUT

PT: 15 min. - **CT:** 25 min.
MODE: Baking - **SERVS:** 2
INGREDIENTS: 2 halibut fillets, 6 oz. each

- 2 Tbls chermoula paste
- 1 Tbls olive oil
- Fresh cilantro leaves for garnish
- Lemon wedges for serving

DIRECTIONS: Pat the halibut dry and spread chermoula paste evenly over fillets

- Drizzle with olive oil and bake in a preheated oven at 375°F (190°C) until the fish flakes easily
- Garnish with cilantro and serve with lemon wedges

TIPS: Serve over a bed of arugula for added peppery flavor

- Chermoula can be made ahead and stored in the fridge

NUTRITIONAL VALUES: Calories: 220 - Fat: 10g - Carbs: 1g - Protein: 31g - Sugar: 0g

CIOPPINO WITH A TWIST

PT: 20 min. - **CT:** 40 min.
MODE: Simmering - **SERVS:** 6
INGREDIENTS: 12 littleneck clams, scrubbed

- 1 lb. mussels, cleaned and debearded
- 8 large shrimp, peeled and deveined
- 1 lb. cod, cut into pieces
- 1 qt. fish stock
- 1 C. crushed tomatoes
- 1 bulb fennel, diced
- 1 tsp saffron threads
- 2 garlic cloves, minced
- ½ C. flat-leaf parsley, chopped
- ¼ C. EVOO
- Red pepper flakes to taste

DIRECTIONS: Sauté fennel and garlic in EVOO until tender

- Add crushed tomatoes, fish stock, and saffron, bring to a low simmer
- Add clams, mussels, shrimp, and cod until seafood is cooked through
- Stir in parsley and season with red pepper flakes

TIPS: Best served with a slice of gluten-free sourdough to soak up the broth

- The stew can be customized with any firm-fleshed fish

NUTRITIONAL VALUES: Calories: 310 - Fat: 8g - Carbs: 12g - Protein: 38g - Sugar: 3g

PISTACHIO-CRUSTED SALMON

PT: 10 min. - **CT:** 15 min.
MODE: Roasting - **SERVS:** 4
INGREDIENTS: 4 salmon fillets, 5 oz. each

- ½ C. shelled pistachios, chopped
- 2 Tbls Dijon mustard
- 1 Tbls honey
- 1 tsp garlic, minced
- Sea salt to taste
- Fresh dill for garnish

DIRECTIONS: Mix mustard, honey, and garlic, then coat salmon fillets

- Press chopped pistachios onto the fillets
- Roast in a preheated oven at 400°F (204°C) until crust is golden and salmon is cooked through
- Garnish with fresh dill

TIPS: The pistachio crust provides not only flavor but also a delightful crunch

- Leftover crust mixture can be used on chicken breasts

NUTRITIONAL VALUES: Calories: 300 - Fat: 18g - Carbs: 5g - Protein: 29g - Sugar: 4g

TARRAGON-INFUSED ORANGE ROUGHY

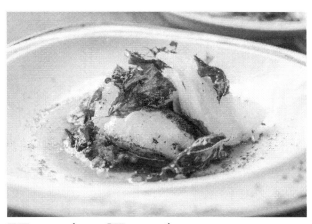

PT: 10 min. - **CT:** 15 min.
MODE: Sautéing - **SERVS:** 4
INGREDIENTS: 4 orange roughy fillets, 4 oz. each

- 1 Tbls fresh tarragon, chopped
- 2 Tbls unsalted butter
- Zest of 1 lemon
- 1 fl. oz. dry white wine
- Sea salt to taste
- Ground black pepper to taste

DIRECTIONS: Season fillets with salt, pepper, and lemon zest

- Melt butter in a skillet, add tarragon and fillets, and cook over medium heat until golden

- Deglaze the pan with white wine and cook until fish is fully cooked

TIPS: Pair with a simple quinoa pilaf for a complete meal

- Any leftover tarragon butter can be used to dress steamed vegetables

NUTRITIONAL VALUES: Calories: 170 - Fat: 5g - Carbs: 0g - Protein: 28g - Sugar: 0g

MISO-GLAZED BLACK COD

PT: 20 min. - **CT:** 10 min.
MODE: Grilling - **SERVS:** 2
INGREDIENTS: 2 black cod fillets, 6 oz. each

- 1 Tbls white miso paste
- 1 Tbls mirin
- 1 Tbls sake
- 1 Tbls soy sauce, reduced sodium
- 1 tsp sugar
- 1 tsp ginger, grated

DIRECTIONS: Mix miso, mirin, sake, soy sauce, sugar, and ginger to make a glaze

- Coat the fillets and let marinate for at least 1 hr.

- Grill on high heat until the glaze caramelizes and fish is cooked through

TIPS: Marinate overnight for more pronounced flavors

- Serve with a side of steamed bok choy for a nutritious meal

NUTRITIONAL VALUES: Calories: 280 - Fat: 12g - Carbs: 9g - Protein: 34g - Sugar: 5g

SHRIMP AND AVOCADO CEVICHE

PT: 30 min. - **CT:** 0 min.
MODE: Marinating - **SERVS:** 6
INGREDIENTS: 1 lb. shrimp, cooked and chopped

- 2 avocados, diced
- 1 red onion, finely chopped
- 1 C. fresh lime juice
- ¼ C. cilantro, chopped
- 1 jalapeño, seeded and minced
- Himalayan pink salt to taste

DIRECTIONS: Combine lime juice, onion, and jalapeño in a bowl

- Add shrimp and let marinate for 20 min., then stir in avocado and cilantro
- Season with Himalayan pink salt

TIPS: The lime juice "cooks" the shrimp, so ensure it's fresh and of high quality

- Can be served in endive cups for a fun presentation

NUTRITIONAL VALUES: Calories: 220 - Fat: 12g - Carbs: 10g - Protein: 20g - Sugar: 2g

Lean and Flavorful Poultry Recipes

Poultry can be a superb vessel for the savory and the succulent, delivering meals that delight the palate while aligning with the virtues of an anti-inflammatory diet. The recipes here are carefully crafted to be lean and robust with flavor. From the exotic aromas of Middle Eastern cuisine to the subtle zest of citrus-infused dishes, each recipe here is a testament to poultry's versatility and its integral role in a health-focused kitchen.

Harissa-Rubbed Grilled Chicken Skewers

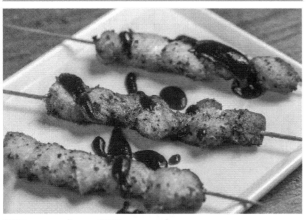

PT: 15 min. - **CT:** 20 min.
MODE: Grilling - **SERVS:** 4
INGREDIENTS: 1 lb. boneless, skinless chicken breast cut into 1-inch pieces

- 2 Tbls harissa paste

- 1 Tbls olive oil

- 1 Tbls apple cider vinegar

- 2 cloves garlic, minced

- 1 tsp ground cumin

- 1 tsp honey

- Salt to taste

- Fresh cilantro leaves for garnish

DIRECTIONS: Trim the chicken, pat dry, and season with salt

- In a bowl, combine harissa, olive oil, vinegar, garlic, cumin, and honey to create a marinade

- Toss chicken pieces in the marinade to coat thoroughly and let sit for 10 minutes

- Thread the chicken onto skewers and grill over medium heat, turning occasionally, until cooked through

TIPS: Serve with a garnish of fresh cilantro for added freshness

- If harissa is too spicy, temper with a bit of yogurt in the marinade

NUTRITIONAL VALUES: Calories: 220

- Fat: 6g - Carbs: 5g - Protein: 35g - Sugar: 3g

Pomegranate Glazed Cornish Hen

PT: 20 min. - **CT:** 1 hr. 15 min.
MODE: Roasting - **SERVS:** 2
INGREDIENTS: 2 Cornish hens, gutted and rinsed

- Salt and black pepper to taste

- 2 Tbls pomegranate molasses

- 1 Tbls olive oil

- 1 Tbls Dijon mustard

- 3 cloves garlic, minced

- 1 tsp fresh thyme leaves

- ½ tsp ground cinnamon

- Pomegranate seeds for garnish

DIRECTIONS: Preheat oven to 375°F (190°C)

- Season the hens with salt and pepper inside and out

- Whisk together pomegranate molasses, olive oil, mustard, garlic, thyme, and cinnamon for the glaze

- Brush the glaze over the hens and roast until the internal temperature reaches 165°F (74°C), basting occasionally

TIPS: Let the hens rest before serving to maintain juiciness

- Garnish with pomegranate seeds for a burst of tartness

NUTRITIONAL VALUES: Calories: 450 - Fat: 22g - Carbs: 15g - Protein: 48g - Sugar: 12g

ZA'ATAR SPICED TURKEY CUTLETS

PT: 10 min. - **CT:** 12 min.
MODE: Sautéing - **SERVS:** 4
INGREDIENTS: 1 lb. turkey breast cutlets

- 3 Tbls za'atar spice mix

- 2 Tbls extra virgin olive oil

- Salt and black pepper to taste

- Lemon wedges for serving

DIRECTIONS: Season turkey cutlets generously with za'atar, salt, and pepper

- Heat olive oil in a large sauté pan over medium-high heat

- Cook cutlets for about 6 minutes per side, or until they have a crisp coating and are cooked through

TIPS: A squeeze of fresh lemon juice before serving adds brightness

- Pair with a crisp salad for a complete meal

NUTRITIONAL VALUES: Calories: 190 - Fat: 5g - Carbs: 0g - Protein: 34g - Sugar: 0g

BALSAMIC FIG CHICKEN THIGHS

PT: 15 min. - **CT:** 40 min.
MODE: Baking - **SERVS:** 4
INGREDIENTS: 8 bone-in, skin-on chicken thighs

- 1 C. fresh figs, quartered

- 2 Tbls balsamic vinegar

- 1 Tbls olive oil

- 1 Tbls raw honey

- 2 sprigs fresh rosemary

- Salt and fresh cracked pepper to taste

DIRECTIONS: Preheat oven to 400°F (200°C)

- Season chicken thighs with salt and pepper and place in a baking dish

- Whisk together balsamic vinegar, olive oil, and honey, and drizzle over chicken

- Tuck figs and rosemary around the thighs and bake until the skin is crispy and the meat is cooked through

TIPS: For a sticky glaze, baste the chicken with pan juices halfway through cooking

- Fresh figs can be substituted with dried figs rehydrated in warm water

NUTRITIONAL VALUES: Calories: 370 - Fat: 20g - Carbs: 18g - Protein: 30g - Sugar: 15g

SESAME-GINGER GROUND TURKEY STIR-FRY

PT: 10 min. - **CT:** 15 min.
MODE: Stir-Frying - **SERVS:** 4
INGREDIENTS: 1 lb. ground turkey

- 1 Tbls sesame oil

- 2 Tbls soy sauce (low sodium)

- 1 Tbls fresh ginger, grated

- 2 cloves garlic, minced

- 1 red bell pepper, thinly sliced

- 1 C. snow peas

- 1 tsp honey

- 1 Tbls sesame seeds

- Scallions for garnish

DIRECTIONS: In a large skillet, heat sesame oil over medium heat

- Add ground turkey and cook until lightly browned

- Stir in soy sauce, ginger, garlic, bell pepper, and snow peas, and cook until vegetables are tender-crisp

- Finish with honey and sprinkle with sesame seeds and scallions

TIPS: Add a spicy kick with a drizzle of sriracha

- Serve over brown rice or quinoa for added fiber

NUTRITIONAL VALUES: Calories: 290 - Fat: 14g - Carbs: 9g - Protein: 32g - Sugar: 5g

ROSEMARY CITRUS ROASTED DUCK BREAST

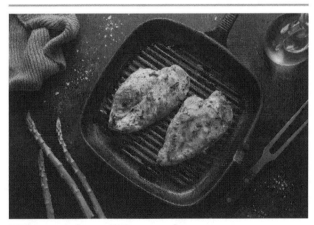

PT: 20 min. - **CT:** 30 min.

MODE: Roasting - **SERVS:** 2

INGREDIENTS: 2 duck breasts, skin scored

- Salt and pepper to taste

- 1 tsp fresh rosemary, finely chopped

- Zest of 1 orange

- 1 Tbls olive oil

- 1 tsp apple cider vinegar

DIRECTIONS: Preheat oven to 400°F (200°C)

- Season duck breasts with salt, pepper, rosemary, and orange zest

- Heat olive oil in an ovenproof skillet over medium-high heat, place duck breasts skin side down and render the fat until skin is golden

- Flip the breasts, add a splash of apple cider vinegar, and roast in the oven until desired doneness

TIPS: Let rest before slicing for juicier meat

- The rendered fat can be used to roast vegetables, adding a rich flavor

NUTRITIONAL VALUES: Calories: 480 - Fat: 40g - Carbs: 1g - Protein: 30g - Sugar: 0g

ANCHO CHILE CHICKEN WITH SWEET POTATOES

PT: 25 min. - **CT:** 45 min.

MODE: Baking - **SERVS:** 4

INGREDIENTS: 4 boneless, skinless chicken breasts

- 1 lb. sweet potatoes, peeled and diced

- 1 Tbls ancho chile powder

- 2 Tbls olive oil

- 1 tsp honey

- 1 tsp smoked paprika

- Juice of 1 lime

- Fresh cilantro for garnish

DIRECTIONS: Preheat oven to 375°F (190°C)

- Toss sweet potatoes with half the olive oil, smoked paprika, and salt, and spread on a baking sheet

- Roast for 20 minutes

- Meanwhile, mix ancho chile powder, remaining olive oil, honey, and lime juice for the chicken marinade

- Coat chicken breasts and place on the baking sheet with sweet potatoes, roasting until the chicken is cooked through

TIPS: Garnish with cilantro for extra color and flavor

- Serve with a dollop of Greek yogurt to balance the chile's warmth

NUTRITIONAL VALUES: Calories: 330 - Fat: 8g - Carbs: 28g - Protein: 36g - Sugar: 7g

MAPLE-MUSTARD SPATCHCOCK CHICKEN

PT: 20 min. - **CT:** 1 hr.

MODE: Roasting - **SERVS:** 4

INGREDIENTS: 1 whole chicken, spatchcocked (backbone removed)

- 3 Tbls Dijon mustard

- 2 Tbls pure maple syrup

- 2 Tbls apple cider vinegar

- 1 Tbls olive oil

- 2 cloves garlic, minced

- Salt and fresh ground pepper to taste

- Fresh thyme for garnish

DIRECTIONS: Preheat oven to 425°F (220°C)

- Season the chicken on both sides with salt and pepper

- Mix together mustard, maple syrup, vinegar, olive oil, and garlic to create a glaze

- Brush the glaze all over the chicken before roasting

- Roast until the skin is crisp and a thermometer reads 165°F (74°C) for the thickest part of the meat

TIPS: Let the chicken rest for 10 minutes for the juices to redistribute

- For a more caramelized crust, broil for the final 2-3 minutes of cooking

NUTRITIONAL VALUES: Calories: 520 - Fat: 31g - Carbs: 15g - Protein: 46g - Sugar: 12g

HARISSA-ROASTED CHICKEN THIGHS

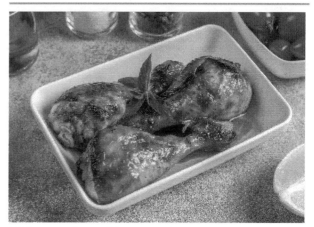

PT: 15 min. - **CT:** 45 min.

MODE: Oven Roasting - **SERVS:** 4

INGREDIENTS: 4 skinless, boneless chicken thighs

- 2 Tbls harissa paste

- 1 Tbls olive oil

- 2 cloves garlic, minced

- 1 tsp ground cumin

- ½ tsp sea salt

- 1 lemon, quartered

DIRECTIONS: Preheat oven to 375°F (190°C)

- In a bowl, mix harissa, olive oil, garlic, cumin, and sea salt to form a paste

- Rub the paste evenly over chicken thighs

- Place thighs on a baking sheet and put in the oven

- Roast for 45 min. or until the chicken is cooked through and has a crisp outer layer

- Serve with a squeeze of fresh lemon juice

TIPS: Avoid overcrowding the pan to ensure chicken cooks evenly and gets a crisp exterior

- For a smokier flavor, add a pinch of smoked paprika to the harissa mixture

NUTRITIONAL VALUES: Calories: 310 - Fat: 18g - Carbs: 3g - Protein: 35g - Sugar: 1g

POULET À L'ESTRAGON

PT: 10 min. - **CT:** 25 min.
MODE: Pan Searing and Simmering - **SERVS:** 4
INGREDIENTS: 1 lb. boneless chicken breasts

- 2 Tbls fresh tarragon, chopped
- 1 Tbls unsalted butter
- 1 shallot, finely chopped
- 1 fl. oz. dry white wine
- ⅔ C. organic chicken stock
- ½ C. Greek yogurt
- Salt and pepper to taste

DIRECTIONS: Season chicken breasts with salt and pepper

- Melt butter in a skillet over medium heat
- Add shallot and cook until translucent
- Increase heat, add chicken, and sear both sides until golden
- Reduce heat, pour in wine, and let simmer for 2 min.
- Add chicken stock and half of the tarragon
- Cover and simmer for 20 min.
- Remove chicken, stir in yogurt and the rest of the tarragon to the sauce
- Drizzle sauce over chicken before serving

TIPS: Use a thermometer to ensure chicken reaches an internal temperature of 165°F (74°C) for safety

- Substitute Greek yogurt with coconut cream for a dairy-free version
- The tarragon leaves can be reserved for garnishing

NUTRITIONAL VALUES: Calories: 215 - Fat: 8g - Carbs: 3g - Protein: 30g - Sugar: 2g

CHICKEN ZOODLES IN THAI GREEN CURRY

PT: 20 min. - **CT:** 15 min.
MODE: Sautéing - **SERVS:** 2
INGREDIENTS: 2 medium zucchinis, spiralized into zoodles

- 1 lb. chicken breast, thinly sliced
- 2 Tbls green curry paste
- 1 can coconut milk
- 1 Tbls fish sauce
- 1 tsp coconut sugar
- Fresh basil and lime wedges for garnish
- Coconut oil for cooking

DIRECTIONS: Heat a skillet with coconut oil over medium-high heat

- Add green curry paste and cook for 1 min.
- Add chicken and sauté until no longer pink
- Pour in coconut milk, fish sauce, and coconut sugar
- Bring to a light simmer and cook for 10 min.
- Add zoodles and heat through for 3-5 min.
- Serve garnished with basil and lime

TIPS: Chicken can be marinated in curry paste for 30 min. ahead for more intensity

- For a vegetarian option, replace chicken with tofu
- Adjust the amount of green curry paste according to spice preference

NUTRITIONAL VALUES: Calories: 400 - Fat: 25g - Carbs: 10g - Protein: 35g - Sugar: 5g

TURMERIC-GINGER CHICKEN STEW

PT: 15 min. - **CT:** 1 hr.
MODE: Slow Cooking - **SERVS:** 6
INGREDIENTS: 2 lbs. chicken thighs, bone-in and skin-on

- 1 inch fresh turmeric, grated

- 1 inch fresh ginger, grated

- 1 yellow onion, chopped

- 3 carrots, peeled and chopped

- 2 C. low-sodium chicken broth

- 1 Tbls apple cider vinegar

- Fresh cilantro for garnish

- Olive oil

- Salt and pepper to taste

DIRECTIONS: Season chicken thighs with salt, pepper, turmeric, and ginger

- Heat olive oil in a large pot over medium-high heat

- Add chicken and brown on both sides

- Transfer chicken onto a plate

- Sauté onions and carrots in the same pot until softened

- Return chicken to the pot, add chicken broth and apple cider vinegar

- Bring to a boil, then cover and simmer on low for 1 hr.

- Garnish with fresh cilantro before serving

TIPS: Adding a pinch of black pepper can enhance turmeric's absorption

- Use a slow cooker for an even softer texture and infusion of flavors

- Skim any excess fat off the top of the stew before serving for a lighter dish

NUTRITIONAL VALUES: Calories: 360 - Fat: 22g - Carbs: 7g - Protein: 32g - Sugar: 3g

SUMAC SPICED CHICKEN SKEWERS

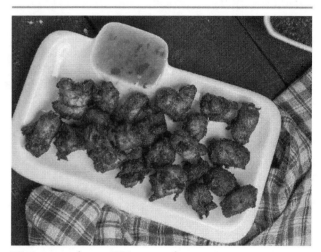

PT: 25 min. - **CT:** 10 min.
MODE: Grilling - **SERVS:** 0
INGREDIENTS: 2 lbs. chicken breast, cut into cubes

- 1 Tbls sumac

- 1 tsp ground coriander

- 2 Tbls olive oil

- 1 lemon, zest and juice

- 2 cloves garlic, minced

- Salt and pepper to taste

- Wooden skewers soaked in water for 30 min.

DIRECTIONS: In a mixing bowl, combine olive oil, lemon zest and juice, sumac, coriander, garlic, salt, and pepper

- Add chicken cubes and marinate for at least 20 min.

- Preheat grill to medium-high heat

- Thread marinated chicken onto skewers

- Grill for 5 min. on each side or until fully cooked

TIPS: Pair with a side of chilled cucumber yogurt dip to balance the tangy flavor of sumac

- If using a stovetop grill pan, make sure it is well-greased to prevent sticking

- Sumac can be replaced with za'atar for a different flavor profile

NUTRITIONAL VALUES: Calories: 205 - Fat: 5g - Carbs: 2g - Protein: 35g - Sugar: 1g

HERBES DE PROVENCE RUBBED CORNISH HEN

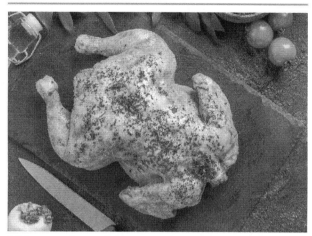

PT: 15 min. - **CT:** 50 min.
MODE: Roasting - **SERVS:** 2
INGREDIENTS: 2 Cornish hens, approximately 1½ lbs. each

- 3 Tbls Herbes de Provence

- 2 cloves garlic, minced

- 1 Tbls olive oil

- 1 lemon, cut into wedges

- Salt and pepper to taste

DIRECTIONS: Preheat oven to 400°F (200°C)

- Pat Cornish hens dry and season inside and out with salt and pepper

- Rub the outside with a mixture of Herbes de Provence, garlic, and olive oil

- Insert lemon wedges into the cavity

- Roast in the oven for 50 min. or until the internal temperature reaches 165°F (74°C)

- Let rest for 10 min. before carving

TIPS: Rubbing the herbes under the skin helps flavor penetrate the meat

- Cornish hens can be stuffed with a mixture of wild rice and mushrooms for a heartier meal

- Leftovers are perfect for a savory chicken salad the following day

NUTRITIONAL VALUES: Calories: 475 - Fat: 27g - Carbs: 3g - Protein: 50g - Sugar: 0g

POLLO PIBIL

PT: 30 min. - **CT:** 1 hr. 30 min.
MODE: Baking and Steaming - **SERVS:** 4
INGREDIENTS: 4 chicken breasts, skinless

- 1 Tbls achiote paste

- 2 Tbls orange juice

- 1 Tbls lime juice

- 1 tsp white vinegar

- ½ C. chicken stock

- 1 red onion, thinly sliced

- 2 Tbls coconut oil

- Banana leaves

- Salt to taste

DIRECTIONS: Preheat oven to 350°F (175°C)

- In a bowl, mix achiote paste, orange juice, lime juice, vinegar, chicken stock, and salt

- Coat chicken breasts with the mixture

- Sauté red onion in coconut oil until soft

- Line a baking dish with banana leaves, leaving enough overhang to cover the chicken

- Place chicken and onions on leaves and fold over to create a parcel

- Bake for 1 hr. 30 min. or until chicken is tender

TIPS: Banana leaves add a subtle flavor and help keep the chicken moist

- Serve with pickled red onions for an authentic Yucatán experience

- Achiote paste is a key ingredient for the traditional Pibil flavor, but in a pinch, you can use a mix of paprika and lemon juice

NUTRITIONAL VALUES: Calories: 280 - Fat: 7g - Carbs: 6g - Protein: 45g - Sugar: 2g

CHICKEN WITH POMEGRANATE AND WALNUTS (FESENJAN)

PT: 15 min. - **CT:** 1 hr.

MODE: Simmering - **SERVS:** 6

INGREDIENTS: 2 lbs. chicken thighs, skinless and boneless

- 1 onion, diced

- 4 C. pomegranate juice

- 1 C. crushed walnuts

- 1 Tbls olive oil

- 2 tsp ground cinnamon

- 1 tsp ground nutmeg

- Salt and freshly ground black pepper to taste

- Fresh pomegranate arils for garnish

DIRECTIONS: Heat olive oil in a large skillet over medium heat

- Sauté the onion until translucent

- Add chicken thighs and brown on all sides

- Pour in pomegranate juice, bring to a simmer

- Add crushed walnuts, cinnamon, nutmeg, salt, and pepper

- Cover and simmer on low heat for 1 hr.

- Uncover and let the sauce reduce until thickened

- Garnish with pomegranate arils before serving

TIPS: Serve with basmati rice to soak up the rich sauce

- Use 100% pure pomegranate juice for maximum flavor and health benefits

- Leftover Fesenjan can be refrigerated and tastes even better the next day as flavors meld

NUTRITIONAL VALUES: Calories: 460 - Fat: 28g - Carbs: 22g - Protein: 30g - Sugar: 16g

TURMERIC-GINGER CHICKEN STIR-FRY

PT: 15 min - **CT:** 10 min

MODE: Stir-Frying - **SERVS:** 2

INGREDIENTS: 2 chicken breasts, thinly sliced

- 1 Tbls fresh turmeric, grated

- 1 Tbls fresh ginger, grated

- 2 tsp coconut oil

- 1 red bell pepper, julienne

- 1 C. snow peas

- 1/2 C. chicken broth, low sodium

- 1 Tbls apple cider vinegar

- 1 tsp raw honey

- Salt to taste

- Fresh cilantro for garnish

DIRECTIONS: Heat coconut oil over medium-high heat in a wok or large pan

- Add turmeric and ginger, cook for 1 min

- Add chicken, stir-fry until golden, about 5 min

- Include bell pepper and snow peas, stir-fry for another 3 min

- Pour in chicken broth, apple cider vinegar, raw honey, and salt, cooking for an additional 2 min

- Garnish with cilantro

TIPS: Opt for organic vegetables to enhance the anti-inflammatory properties

- Pair with brown rice or quinoa for a complete meal

NUTRITIONAL VALUES: Calories: 220 - Fat: 6g - Carbs: 12g - Protein: 30g - Sugar: 5g

POMEGRANATE GLAZED TURKEY CUTLETS

PT: 10 min - **CT:** 15 min
MODE: Pan-searing - **SERVS:** 4
INGREDIENTS: 4 turkey cutlets, 1/4 inch thick

- Salt and pepper to taste
- 1 Tbls olive oil
- 1/2 C. pomegranate juice
- 1 Tbls balsamic vinegar
- 1 tsp Dijon mustard
- 1 garlic clove, minced
- 1 tsp arrowroot starch
- Pomegranate arils for garnish

DIRECTIONS: Season cutlets with salt and pepper

- Heat olive oil over medium-high heat in a skillet
- Pan-sear cutlets until just cooked through, about 4 min per side, remove and set aside
- In the same skillet, combine pomegranate juice, balsamic vinegar, Dijon mustard, and garlic, simmer until reduced by half
- Whisk arrowroot starch with a little water, then stir into sauce, simmer until thickened
- Drizzle sauce over cutlets, garnish with pomegranate arils

TIPS: Arrowroot starch serves as a phenomenal thickening agent that does not interfere with the anti-inflammatory profile

- A scatter of fresh mint leaves can add an additional layer of freshness

NUTRITIONAL VALUES: Calories: 200 - Fat: 5g - Carbs: 10g - Protein: 28g - Sugar: 6g

MEDITERRANEAN CHICKEN KABOBS

PT: 25 min - **CT:** 15 min
MODE: Grilling - **SERVS:** 4
INGREDIENTS: 2 lb. chicken breast, cubed

- 1 Tbls extra virgin olive oil
- 2 tsp za'atar spice mix
- 1 lemon, juiced and zested
- 2 garlic cloves, minced
- 1 red onion, cut into chunks
- 1 C. cherry tomatoes
- 1 C. zucchini, thickly sliced
- Salt and pepper to taste

DIRECTIONS: Marinate chicken with olive oil, za'atar, lemon juice, zest, garlic, salt, and pepper for 20 min

- Preheat grill to medium-high heat, 375°F (190°C)
- Thread chicken, onion, tomatoes, and zucchini onto skewers
- Grill for about 15 min, turning occasionally until chicken is cooked through

TIPS: Marinating time is essential for robust flavor infusion

- Serve with a drizzle of tahini for extra creaminess
- Keep lemon wedges handy to squeeze over the kabobs before serving for extra zest

NUTRITIONAL VALUES: Calories: 310 - Fat: 9g - Carbs: 8g - Protein: 48g - Sugar: 4g

CILANTRO-LIME TURKEY MEATBALLS

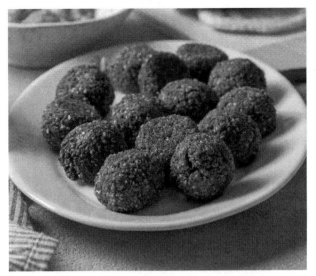

PT: 20 min - **CT:** 30 min
MODE: Baking - **SERVS:** 5
INGREDIENTS: 1 lb. ground turkey

- 1/4 C. almond flour

- 1 egg, beaten

- 1/4 C. fresh cilantro, finely chopped

- 1 lime, juiced and zested

- 1 tsp ground cumin

- 1/2 tsp smoked paprika

- 1/4 tsp sea salt

- 2 Tbls avocado oil

DIRECTIONS: Preheat oven to 400°F (200°C)

- Combine turkey, almond flour, egg, cilantro, lime juice, zest, cumin, smoked paprika, salt

- Form into 1-inch meatballs

- Place on a baking sheet brushed with avocado oil

- Bake for 30 min or until golden and cooked through

TIPS: Replacing bread crumbs with almond flour adds a nutritious twist and keeps the meatballs gluten-free

- Squeeze additional lime juice over the meatballs before serving for a tangy punch

NUTRITIONAL VALUES: Calories: 180 - Fat: 10g - Carbs: 4g - Protein: 20g - Sugar: 1g

HERB-ROASTED CHICKEN THIGHS

PT: 15 min - **CT:** 45 min
MODE: Roasting - **SERVS:** 6
INGREDIENTS: 6 bone-in, skin-on chicken thighs

- 2 Tbls avocado oil

- 1 Tbls fresh rosemary, minced

- 1 Tbls fresh thyme, minced

- 2 tsp fresh oregano, minced

- 4 garlic cloves, minced

- Salt and cracked black pepper to taste

DIRECTIONS: Preheat oven to 425°F (220°C)

- Rub chicken thighs with avocado oil, rosemary, thyme, oregano, garlic, salt, and pepper

- Place on a roasting tray

- Roast for about 45 min or until skin is crispy and meat is cooked through

TIPS: Herbs can be swapped according to seasonal availability

- Reserve pan juices to drizzle on top of a side of mashed cauliflower

NUTRITIONAL VALUES: Calories: 400 - Fat: 28g - Carbs: 2g - Protein: 34g - Sugar: 0g

SMOKY CHICKEN AND QUINOA STEW

PT: 10 min - **CT:** 25 min
MODE: Simmering - **SERVS:** 4
INGREDIENTS: 1 Tbls coconut oil

- 1 small onion, diced

- 2 garlic cloves, minced

- 1 tsp smoked paprika

- 1/2 tsp cayenne pepper

- 2 cups shredded cooked chicken breast

- 1 qt. chicken stock, low sodium

- 1 C. cooked quinoa

- 1/2 C. diced fire-roasted tomatoes

- Sea salt and ground black pepper to taste

DIRECTIONS: Heat coconut oil in a large pot over medium heat

- Sauté onion and garlic until translucent

- Add smoked paprika, cayenne, and stir for 1 min

- Add chicken, stock, quinoa, and tomatoes

- Season with salt and pepper

- Bring to a boil, then simmer for 20 min

TIPS: This stew can be made in advance and freezes well

- Opt for homemade stock to control sodium and quality

- A dollop of Greek yogurt can add creaminess and a probiotic boost

NUTRITIONAL VALUES: Calories: 275 - Fat: 7g - Carbs: 25g - Protein: 30g - Sugar: 4g

SIDES AND APPETIZERS: TASTY AND HEALTHY BITES

Sides and appetizers offer a delightful gateway into the world of anti-inflammatory eating, presenting a cornucopia of flavors and nutrients. The recipes here are crafted to tantalize the palate while keeping health at the forefront. We'll explore unique combinations that are both heartwarming and healing, stimulating the senses without compromising wellness. Each dish is a step towards embracing a lifestyle that combats inflammation and cherishes the joy of eating.

CHARRED SHISHITO PEPPERS WITH LEMON AIOLI

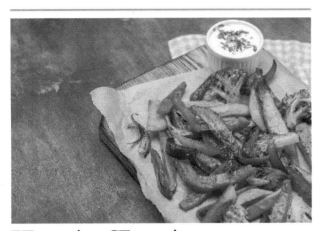

PT: 10 min. - **CT:** 10 min.
MODE: Grilling - **SERVS:** 4
INGREDIENTS: 8 oz. shishito peppers

- 1 Tbls extra virgin olive oil
- Salt to taste
- 1 small garlic clove, minced
- ½ C. silken tofu
- 1 Tbls lemon zest
- 2 Tbls lemon juice
- 1 Tbls apple cider vinegar
- Freshly ground black pepper to taste

DIRECTIONS: Toss shishito peppers with olive oil and salt

- Grill over medium heat, turning frequently, until blistered and slightly charred

- For the aioli, blend the minced garlic, silken tofu, lemon zest, lemon juice, and apple cider vinegar until smooth, season with salt and black pepper

- Serve peppers with aioli dipping sauce

TIPS: Opt for grilling outdoors to enhance the smoky flavor of peppers

- If indoor grilling, use a well-ventilated area or a grill pan

- Aioli can be stored in the refrigerator for up to 5 days

NUTRITIONAL VALUES: Calories: 70 - Fat: 4g - Carbs: 7g - Protein: 2g - Sugar: 3g

JICAMA FRIES WITH CILANTRO LIME DRIZZLE

PT: 15 min. - **CT:** 25 min.
MODE: Baking - **SERVS:** 4
INGREDIENTS: 1 medium jicama, peeled and cut into fries

- 2 Tbls avocado oil
- 1 tsp ground cumin
- 1 tsp smoked paprika
- Salt to taste
- ¼ C. chopped fresh cilantro
- Juice of 1 lime
- 1 Tbls nutritional yeast
- 1 small garlic clove, minced

DIRECTIONS: Preheat oven to 425°F (218°C)

- Toss jicama with 1 Tbls avocado oil, cumin, smoked paprika, salt, and spread on a baking sheet

- Bake until edges are crisp, about 25 min
- Whisk together 1 Tbls avocado oil, cilantro, lime juice, nutritional yeast, and minced garlic for the drizzle
- Serve fries topped with cilantro lime drizzle

TIPS: Jicama can be replaced with turnips for similar results

- Nutritional yeast adds a cheese-like flavor and additional nutrients
- Leftover cilantro lime drizzle makes an excellent salad dressing

NUTRITIONAL VALUES: Calories: 120 - Fat: 7g - Carbs: 13g - Protein: 2g - Sugar: 3g

SPICED MOROCCAN CARROT DIP

PT: 20 min. - **CT:** 45 min.
MODE: Baking - **SERVS:** 6
INGREDIENTS: 1 lb. carrots, peeled and diced

- 2 Tbls extra virgin olive oil
- 1 tsp ground coriander
- ½ tsp ground cumin
- ¼ tsp ground cinnamon
- ¼ tsp cayenne pepper
- Salt and ground black pepper to taste
- 2 Tbls tahini
- 2 Tbls orange juice
- 1 garlic clove
- 1 tsp fresh ginger, grated

DIRECTIONS: Preheat oven to 400°F (204°C)

- Toss carrots with 1 Tbls olive oil, coriander, cumin, cinnamon, cayenne, salt, and pepper
- Roast until tender, about 45 min

- Blend roasted carrots, remaining olive oil, tahini, orange juice, garlic, and ginger until smooth

TIPS: Serve with vegetable crudites or gluten-free crackers

- Can be enriched with a swirl of harissa for extra heat
- Refrigerate to allow flavors to meld more deeply overnight

NUTRITIONAL VALUES: Calories: 98 - Fat: 5g - Carbs: 12g - Protein: 2g - Sugar: 5g

ZA'ATAR SPICED CHICKPEA POPPERS

PT: 10 min. - **CT:** 30 min.
MODE: Roasting - **SERVS:** 4
INGREDIENTS: 2 C. chickpeas, cooked and drained

- 1 Tbls za'atar seasoning
- 1 Tbls extra virgin olive oil
- Salt to taste

DIRECTIONS: Preheat oven to 375°F (190°C)

- Pat chickpeas dry and toss with za'atar seasoning, olive oil, and salt
- Spread on a baking sheet and roast until crispy, about 30 min

TIPS: Za'atar can be made at home by combining dried thyme, toasted sesame seeds, and sumac

- Serve as a crunchy topping on soups and salads
- Store in an airtight container to maintain crispness

NUTRITIONAL VALUES: Calories: 134 - Fat: 4g - Carbs: 19g - Protein: 6g - Sugar: 3g

CHILLED EDAMAME GAZPACHO

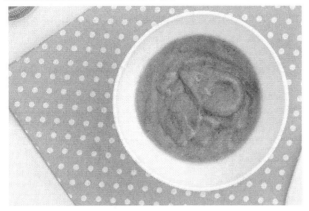

PT: 20 min. - **CT:** 0 min.
MODE: Blending - **SERVS:** 4
INGREDIENTS: 2 C. shelled edamame

- 1 cucumber, peeled and chopped
- 1 green bell pepper, chopped
- 1 small white onion, chopped
- 2 cloves garlic
- 1 avocado
- Juice of 1 lime
- 2 C. vegetable broth
- Salt and ground black pepper to taste
- Fresh parsley for garnish

DIRECTIONS: Blend edamame, cucumber, bell pepper, onion, garlic, avocado, lime juice, and vegetable broth until smooth

- Season with salt and pepper
- Chill for an hour before serving
- Garnish with parsley

TIPS: Gazpacho can be served as a refreshing dip

- For a spicier version, add a jalapeño to the blend
- Use homemade vegetable broth for a richer flavor profile

NUTRITIONAL VALUES: Calories: 180 - Fat: 9g - Carbs: 17g - Protein: 11g - Sugar: 5g

CUMIN-INFUSED BEET HUMMUS

PT: 15 min. - **CT:** 0 min.
MODE: Blending - **SERVS:** 6
INGREDIENTS: 15 oz. can of beets, drained and rinsed

- 1 C. cooked chickpeas
- 2 Tbls tahini
- 2 Tbls extra virgin olive oil
- Juice of 1 lemon
- 1 tsp ground cumin
- 1 small garlic clove
- Salt and ground black pepper to taste

DIRECTIONS: Blend beets, chickpeas, tahini, olive oil, lemon juice, cumin, garlic, salt, and pepper until smooth and creamy

TIPS: Serve with an array of colorful vegetable sticks for dipping

- For a smokier flavor, use roasted beets instead of canned
- Garnish with sesame seeds and a drizzle of olive oil for added texture and taste

NUTRITIONAL VALUES: Calories: 102 - Fat: 5g - Carbs: 12g - Protein: 3g - Sugar: 5g

TURMERIC CAULIFLOWER BITES

PT: 15 min. - **CT:** 20 min.
MODE: Baking - **SERVS:** 4
INGREDIENTS: 1 head of cauliflower, cut into bite-sized florets

- 1 Tbls coconut oil, melted
- 1 tsp turmeric
- ½ tsp garlic powder
- Salt and ground black pepper to taste
- 2 Tbls almond flour
- Fresh cilantro for garnish

DIRECTIONS: Preheat oven to 450°F (232°C)

- Toss cauliflower florets with coconut oil, turmeric, garlic powder, salt, and pepper

- Sprinkle with almond flour and toss again to coat
- Bake until golden and tender, about 20 min
- Garnish with fresh cilantro

TIPS: Turmeric can stain surfaces, so consider using gloves and protective coverings

- Almond flour can be substituted with coconut flour for a different flavor profile
- These bites can also be air-fried for a crisper texture

NUTRITIONAL VALUES: Calories: 77 - Fat: 4g - Carbs: 9g - Protein: 3g - Sugar: 3g

BALSAMIC BRUSCHETTA ON SWEET POTATO ROUNDS

PT: 20 min. - **CT:** 15 min.
MODE: Baking - **SERVS:** 6
INGREDIENTS: 2 large sweet potatoes, sliced into ¼-inch rounds

- 2 Tbls balsamic vinegar
- 1 pt. cherry tomatoes, quartered
- 1 small red onion, finely chopped
- ¼ C. fresh basil leaves, chopped
- 1 Tbls extra virgin olive oil
- Salt and ground black pepper to taste

DIRECTIONS: Preheat oven to 425°F (218°C)

- Arrange sweet potato rounds on a baking sheet, bake until tender, about 15 min
- Mix tomatoes, red onion, basil, balsamic vinegar, olive oil, salt, and pepper
- Top sweet potato rounds with tomato mixture

TIPS: Using a mandolin ensures uniform slices of sweet potato

- The bruschetta topping can also be enjoyed on its own as a salad

- Drizzle with a reduced balsamic glaze for a more intense flavor

NUTRITIONAL VALUES: Calories: 113 - Fat: 2g - Carbs: 21g - Protein: 2g - Sugar: 7g

CURRIED CAULIFLOWER FLORETS

PT: 10 min - **CT:** 25 min
MODE: Roasting - **SERVS:** 6
INGREDIENTS: 1 head cauliflower, cut into florets

- 1 Tbls extra virgin olive oil
- 1 tsp turmeric
- 1 tsp garam masala
- 1/2 tsp ginger, ground
- 1/2 tsp garlic powder
- 1/4 tsp cayenne pepper
- Salt to taste

DIRECTIONS: Preheat oven to 425°F (220°C)

- Toss cauliflower with olive oil, turmeric, garam masala, ginger, garlic powder, cayenne pepper, and salt
- Spread on a baking sheet and roast until golden and tender

TIPS: Sprinkle with fresh cilantro for a burst of color

- Pair with a cooling yogurt dip to mellow the spice

NUTRITIONAL VALUES: Calories: 70 - Fat: 3.5g - Carbs: 9g - Protein: 3g - Sugar: 3g

AVOCADO AND EDAMAME SMASH

PT: 15 min - **CT:** 0 min
MODE: No Cooking - **SERVS:** 4
INGREDIENTS: 2 ripe avocados, pitted and scooped

- 1 C. edamame, shelled and cooked
- 1 Tbls lime juice
- 1/2 tsp chili flakes

- 1 Tbls cilantro, chopped

- Salt and pepper to taste

DIRECTIONS: Mash avocados and edamame together in a bowl

- Stir in lime juice, chili flakes, cilantro, salt, and pepper until well combined

TIPS: Top with toasted sesame seeds for crunch

- Serve with endive leaves for a low-carb option

NUTRITIONAL VALUES: Calories: 230

- Fat: 19g - Carbs: 12g - Protein: 8g - Sugar: 1g

SPICED BEETROOT AND QUINOA TABBOULEH

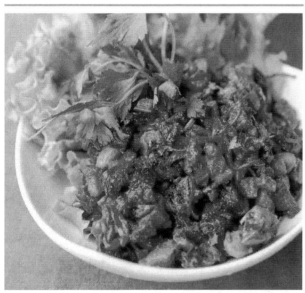

PT: 20 min - **CT:** 0 min

MODE: No Cooking - **SERVS:** 4

INGREDIENTS: 2 C. cooked quinoa

- 1 C. beetroot, grated

- 1/2 C. cucumber, diced

- 1/4 C. red onion, finely chopped

- 2 Tbls fresh parsley, chopped

- 2 Tbls fresh mint, chopped

- 1 Tbls olive oil

- 2 Tbls lemon juice

- 1/2 tsp cumin

- 1/2 tsp coriander

- Salt and pepper to taste

DIRECTIONS: Combine quinoa, beetroot, cucumber, red onion, parsley, and mint in a bowl

- In a separate bowl, whisk together olive oil, lemon juice, cumin, coriander, salt, and pepper

- Pour dressing over quinoa mixture and toss to combine

TIPS: Serve chilled for a refreshing bite

- Garnish with lemon zest for an added zing

NUTRITIONAL VALUES: Calories: 180

- Fat: 4g - Carbs: 30g - Protein: 6g - Sugar: 5g

BALSAMIC ROASTED CARROTS

PT: 10 min - **CT:** 30 min

MODE: Roasting - **SERVS:** 4

INGREDIENTS: 8 medium carrots, peeled and sliced lengthwise

- 2 Tbls balsamic vinegar

- 1 Tbls honey

- 1 Tbls olive oil

- 1/2 tsp thyme, dried

- Salt and pepper to taste

DIRECTIONS: Preheat oven to 400°F (200°C)

- Whisk together balsamic vinegar, honey, olive oil, thyme, salt, and pepper

- Toss carrots in the mixture and spread on a baking sheet

- Roast until tender and caramelized

TIPS: Toss with fresh parsley before serving for a fresh contrast

- Drizzle a touch more balsamic for added tang

NUTRITIONAL VALUES: Calories: 120 - Fat: 5g - Carbs: 18g - Protein: 1g - Sugar: 12g

ZESTY LIME AND CHIA SEED HUMMUS

PT: 15 min - **CT:** 0 min
MODE: No Cooking - **SERVS:** 8
INGREDIENTS: 1 C. chickpeas, cooked and drained

- 1 Tbls chia seeds
- 2 Tbls lime juice
- 2 garlic cloves
- 1/4 C. tahini
- 1/4 C. extra virgin olive oil
- Salt and pepper to taste

DIRECTIONS: Blend chickpeas, chia seeds, lime juice, garlic, tahini, and olive oil in a food processor until smooth

- Season with salt and pepper to taste

TIPS: Add a swirl of chili oil for kick

- Refrigerate for at least 1 hr before serving to allow flavors to meld

NUTRITIONAL VALUES: Calories: 190 - Fat: 13g - Carbs: 16g - Protein: 6g - Sugar: 2g

SESAME GINGER EGGPLANT STICKS

PT: 15 min - **CT:** 20 min
MODE: Baking - **SERVS:** 6
INGREDIENTS: 2 large eggplants, cut into sticks

- 2 Tbls sesame oil
- 2 Tbls tamari sauce
- 1 Tbls ginger, freshly grated
- 1 garlic clove, minced
- Sesame seeds for garnish
- Salt to taste

DIRECTIONS: Preheat oven to 375°F (190°C)

- Whisk together sesame oil, tamari sauce, ginger, and garlic

- Toss eggplant sticks in the mixture and spread on a baking sheet
- Bake until tender and slightly crisp
- Sprinkle with sesame seeds

TIPS: Serve with a side of wasabi mayo for an extra kick

- Allow to cool slightly before serving to intensify flavors

NUTRITIONAL VALUES: Calories: 110 - Fat: 7g - Carbs: 10g - Protein: 2g - Sugar: 6g

SUN-DRIED TOMATO AND OLIVE TAPENADE

PT: 10 min - **CT:** 0 min
MODE: Mixing - **SERVS:** 5
INGREDIENTS: 1/2 C. sun-dried tomatoes, chopped

- 1/2 C. Kalamata olives, pitted and chopped
- 1 Tbls capers, drained
- 2 Tbls parsley, fresh and chopped
- 1 Tbls extra virgin olive oil
- 1 tsp lemon zest
- 1 garlic clove, minced
- Salt and pepper to taste

DIRECTIONS: Mix sun-dried tomatoes, olives, capers, parsley, olive oil, lemon zest, and minced garlic in a bowl

- Season with salt and pepper to taste

TIPS: Serve on whole-grain toast points

- Drizzle with a little more olive oil before serving for a richer flavor

NUTRITIONAL VALUES: Calories: 90 - Fat: 7g - Carbs: 6g - Protein: 1g - Sugar: 3g

HERB-INFUSED MUSHROOM PÂTÉ

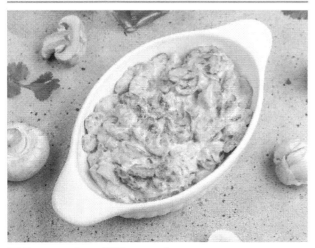

PT: 20 min - **CT:** 15 min
MODE: Sautéing - **SERVS:** 6
INGREDIENTS: 1 lb. mixed mushrooms, chopped

  - 1/4 C. shallots, finely diced
  - 2 Tbls mixed fresh herbs (thyme, parsley, rosemary), chopped
  - 2 Tbls extra virgin olive oil
  - 1/4 C. walnuts, toasted
  - 1/2 tsp apple cider vinegar
  - Salt and pepper to taste

DIRECTIONS: Sauté mushrooms and shallots in olive oil until soft

  - Add herbs and cook for an additional minute
  - Let cool, then blend with walnuts and apple cider vinegar in a food processor until smooth
  - Season with salt and pepper

TIPS: Serve with gluten-free crackers

  - Garnish with additional herbs for a decorative touch

NUTRITIONAL VALUES: Calories: 130 - Fat: 11g - Carbs: 6g - Protein: 4g - Sugar: 2g

SPICED BEET AND LENTIL SALAD

PT: 20 min. - **CT:** 0 min.
MODE: No Cooking - **SERVS:** 4
INGREDIENTS: 2 C. red beets, roasted and cubed

  - 1 C. green lentils, cooked
  - ½ red onion, thinly sliced
  - ¼ C. fresh mint, chopped
  - 3 Tbls extra virgin olive oil
  - 1 Tbls apple cider vinegar
  - 1 tsp ground cumin
  - ¼ tsp ground coriander
  - Salt and pepper to taste

DIRECTIONS: Combine all ingredients in a large bowl

  - Toss gently to mix flavors
  - Let it sit for 10 min. before serving

TIPS: Serve with a dollop of Greek yogurt for added creaminess

  - Can be prepared ahead and refrigerated
  - Use pre-cooked lentils for a quicker prep time

NUTRITIONAL VALUES: Calories: 220 - Fat: 6g - Carbs: 35g - Protein: 9g - Sugar: 9g

CHARRED EDAMAME WITH SEA SALT AND CITRUS ZEST

PT: 5 min. - **CT:** 5 min.
MODE: Sautéing - **SERVS:** 4
INGREDIENTS: 2 C. edamame in pods

  - 1 Tbls olive oil
  - Zest of 1 lemon
  - Zest of 1 orange
  - Coarse sea salt to taste

DIRECTIONS: Heat olive oil in a skillet over high heat

  - Add edamame and cook until charred in spots

- Remove from heat and toss with lemon and orange zest

- Season with sea salt

TIPS: Edamame can be eaten warm or cold

- Perfect for stimulating the appetite before dinner

- Zests can be replaced by lime or grapefruit for variety

NUTRITIONAL VALUES: Calories: 190 - Fat: 9g - Carbs: 13g - Protein: 17g - Sugar: 3g

CRISPY TURMERIC CAULIFLOWER FLORETS

PT: 10 min. - **CT:** 25 min.

MODE: Baking - **SERVS:** 6

INGREDIENTS: 1 large head cauliflower, cut into florets

- 2 Tbls avocado oil

- 1 Tbls turmeric powder

- ½ tsp garlic powder

- ½ tsp smoked paprika

- Salt to taste

DIRECTIONS: Preheat oven to 425°F (218°C)

- Toss cauliflower florets with avocado oil, turmeric, garlic powder, smoked paprika, and salt

- Spread on a baking sheet and bake until crisp and golden

TIPS: Turmeric may stain, use gloves if desired

- Pair with a cucumber yogurt dip for a refreshing contrast

- Opt for a silicone baking mat for a non-stick surface and easy cleanup

NUTRITIONAL VALUES: Calories: 77 - Fat: 5g - Carbs: 8g - Protein: 3g - Sugar: 3g

SESAME GINGER BOK CHOY

PT: 15 min. - **CT:** 10 min.

MODE: Steaming - **SERVS:** 4

INGREDIENTS: 4 baby bok choy, halved lengthwise

- 1 Tbls sesame oil

- 2 tsp ginger, freshly grated

- 1 garlic clove, minced

- 1 tsp soy sauce (gluten-free if necessary)

- 1 tsp sesame seeds

- Salt and pepper to taste

DIRECTIONS: Steam bok choy until tender-crisp

- Heat sesame oil in a pan and sauté ginger and garlic until fragrant

- Stir in steamed bok choy and soy sauce

- Cook for an additional minute

- Sprinkle with sesame seeds

TIPS: Steam larger bok choy a few minutes longer for desired tenderness

- Opt for low-sodium soy sauce to control salt intake

- Garnish with scallions for an extra pop of flavor

NUTRITIONAL VALUES: Calories: 60 - Fat: 5g - Carbs: 4g - Protein: 2g - Sugar: 1g

Stuffed Bell Peppers with Quinoa and Kale

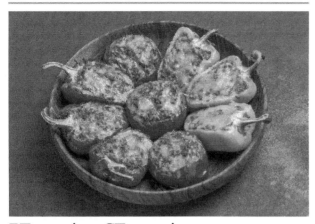

PT: 15 min. - **CT:** 30 min.
MODE: Baking - **SERVS:** 6
INGREDIENTS: 6 bell peppers, tops cut and seeds removed

- 1 C. quinoa, cooked
- 1 C. kale, chopped and steamed
- ½ C. cherry tomatoes, halved
- ⅓ C. feta cheese, crumbled
- ¼ C. pine nuts, toasted
- 2 Tbls balsamic vinegar
- 1 Tbls extra virgin olive oil
- 1 tsp dried oregano
- Salt and pepper to taste

DIRECTIONS: Preheat oven to 350°F (177°C)

- Mix quinoa, kale, tomatoes, feta cheese, pine nuts, balsamic vinegar, and seasonings
- Stuff mixture into bell peppers
- Drizzle with olive oil
- Bake until peppers are tender

TIPS: Can be served cold as a salad

- Replace feta with nutritional yeast for a dairy-free option
- Use a variety of colored peppers for a vibrant presentation

NUTRITIONAL VALUES: Calories: 256
- Fat: 10g - Carbs: 34g - Protein: 9g - Sugar: 7g

Sweet Potato Hummus

PT: 15 min. - **CT:** 45 min.
MODE: Baking - **SERVS:** 10
INGREDIENTS: 2 medium sweet potatoes, peeled and diced

- 1 C. chickpeas, cooked
- 2 Tbls tahini
- 2 garlic cloves, minced
- 2 Tbls lemon juice
- 1 tsp paprika
- ¼ tsp cayenne pepper
- Salt to taste

DIRECTIONS: Preheat oven to 400°F (204°C)

- Roast sweet potatoes until tender
- Blend roasted sweet potatoes, chickpeas, tahini, garlic, lemon juice, paprika, cayenne, and salt until smooth

TIPS: Serve with sliced cucumber and carrots for dipping

- Drizzle with olive oil and a sprinkle of paprika to garnish
- Can be used as a spread for wraps or sandwiches

NUTRITIONAL VALUES: Calories: 123 - Fat: 3g - Carbs: 21g - Protein: 4g - Sugar: 5g

SOUPS RECIPES FOR ALL SEASONS

In this chapter, we dive into a symphony of soothing soups, perfect for any season. From the delicate flavors of a springtime broth to the hearty embrace of a winter stew, these anti-inflammatory recipes offer both nourishment and comfort. As perennial as the changing leaves or the first snowfall, there's a soup here to warm the soul, alleviate pain, and invigorate the immune system with each delightful spoonful.

GOLDEN TURMERIC CHICKPEA SOUP

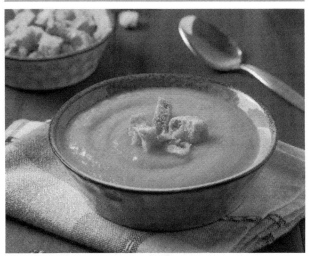

PT: 20 min - **CT:** 35 min
MODE: Simmering - **SERVS:** 4
INGREDIENTS: 1 Tbls extra virgin olive oil

- 1 medium yellow onion, diced
- 2 cloves garlic, minced
- 1 Tbls fresh ginger, grated
- 1 Tbls ground turmeric
- 1 tsp cumin
- 4 C. low-sodium vegetable broth
- 1 C. water
- 1 C. chickpeas, cooked
- 2 C. kale, de-stemmed and chopped
- 1 C. carrots, sliced
- Salt and pepper to taste
- Fresh cilantro for garnish

DIRECTIONS: Heat olive oil in a large soup pot over medium heat
- Sauté onion until translucent
- Add garlic and ginger, cook for 1 min
- Stir in turmeric and cumin
- Add broth, water, chickpeas, kale, carrots, salt, and pepper
- Bring to a simmer, cover, and cook for 35 min
- Garnish with cilantro before serving

TIPS: Serve with a squeeze of lemon for added zest
- Pair with whole grain toast for a filling meal

NUTRITIONAL VALUES: Calories: 210 - Fat: 6g - Carbs: 30g - Protein: 9g - Sugar: 5g

PUMPKIN AND WHITE BEAN SOUP

PT: 20 min - **CT:** 1 hr
MODE: Stovetop - **SERVS:** 6
INGREDIENTS: 2 Tbls olive oil
- 1 small pumpkin, peeled and cubed
- 1 onion, diced
- 3 garlic cloves, minced
- 4 C. vegetable broth
- 1 C. white beans, cooked
- 1 tsp ground cinnamon
- 1/2 tsp ground nutmeg
- Salt and pepper to taste
- Fresh sage for garnish

DIRECTIONS: Heat olive oil in a large pot
- Sauté pumpkin, onion, and garlic until pumpkin is soft

- Add broth, beans, cinnamon, and nutmeg, bring to a boil then simmer for 45 min

- Blend until smooth

- Season with salt and pepper

- Serve garnished with sage

TIPS: Serve with a drizzle of maple syrup for sweetness

- Top with roasted pecans for added crunch

NUTRITIONAL VALUES: Calories: 180 - Fat: 5g - Carbs: 30g - Protein: 7g - Sugar: 6g

HEIRLOOM TOMATO AND WHITE BEAN SOUP

PT: 10 min - **CT:** 25 min
MODE: Simmering - **SERVS:** 6
INGREDIENTS: 4 C. heirloom tomatoes, chopped

- 2 C. white beans, cooked

- 1 Tbls olive oil

- 1 qt. vegetable stock

- 1 bay leaf

- 2 tsp fresh thyme leaves

- 1 Tbls balsamic reduction

- Salt and cracked pepper to taste

DIRECTIONS: Heat olive oil in a large soup pot over medium heat

- Add chopped heirloom tomatoes and cook for 5 min

- Stir in white beans, vegetable stock, bay leaf, and thyme leaves

- Simmer for 20 min

- Remove the bay leaf

- Drizzle with balsamic reduction, season with salt and pepper

TIPS: Top with a garnish of microgreens for a burst of flavor

- Serve with crusty whole grain bread

NUTRITIONAL VALUES: Calories: 180 - Fat: 3g - Carbs: 30g - Protein: 10g - Sugar: 4g

MISO MUSHROOM IMMUNITY BROTH

PT: 15 min - **CT:** 30 min
MODE: Simmering - **SERVS:** 4
INGREDIENTS: 4 C. mushroom broth

- 1 Tbls miso paste

- 1 C. shiitake mushrooms, thinly sliced

- 1 tsp grated ginger

- 2 garlic cloves, thinly sliced

- 1 Tbls Tamari sauce

- 1 tsp toasted sesame oil

- 2 scallions, chopped

- Tofu cubes, optional

- Seaweed, cut into strips

DIRECTIONS: Warm the mushroom broth in a soup pot over medium heat

- Whisk in miso paste until fully dissolved

- Add shiitake mushrooms, ginger, garlic, Tamari sauce, and simmer for 30 min

- Stir in toasted sesame oil

- Top with scallions, tofu if using, and seaweed

TIPS: A pinch of chilli flakes adds a gentle heat

- Incorporate baked tofu for added protein

- Pour over cooked rice noodles for a heartier dish

NUTRITIONAL VALUES: Calories: 100 - Fat: 4g - Carbs: 12g - Protein: 5g - Sugar: 2g

SPICY CARROT AND LENTIL CREAM

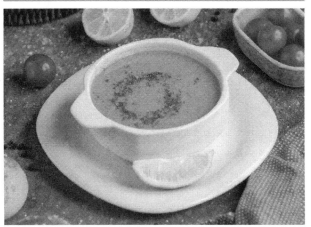

PT: 15 min - **CT:** 40 min
MODE: Simmering - **SERVS:** 6
INGREDIENTS: 2 Tbls coconut oil
 - 1 lb. carrots, peeled and chopped
 - 1 C. red lentils
 - 1 qt. low-sodium vegetable broth
 - 1 Tbls ground coriander
 - 1 tsp smoked paprika
 - 1/2 tsp cayenne pepper
 - 1/2 C. coconut milk
 - Salt to taste
 - Fresh parsley for garnish
DIRECTIONS: Melt coconut oil in a large pot over medium heat
 - Add carrots and cook until they start to soften
 - Stir in red lentils, vegetable broth, coriander, smoked paprika, and cayenne pepper
 - Bring to boil, then simmer for 40 min until lentils are tender
 - Blend until smooth, stir in coconut milk, and season with salt
 - Garnish with parsley
TIPS: Serve with a dollop of Greek yogurt to tame the heat if needed

 - Top with toasted pumpkin seeds for crunch
NUTRITIONAL VALUES: Calories: 190 - Fat: 6g - Carbs: 28g - Protein: 8g - Sugar: 5g

ROASTED BEETROOT AND FENNEL SOUP

PT: 15 min - **CT:** 1 hr
MODE: Roasting and Blending - **SERVS:** 4
INGREDIENTS: 3 medium beetroots, peeled and diced
 - 1 bulb fennel, sliced
 - 2 Tbls avocado oil
 - 1/2 tsp sea salt
 - 4 C. vegetable broth
 - 1 Tbls apple cider vinegar
 - 1/2 tsp ground black pepper
 - 2 Tbls coconut cream
 - Dill fronds for garnish
DIRECTIONS: Toss beetroots and fennel with avocado oil and sea salt, spread on a baking sheet, and roast at 400°F (200°C) for 45 min
 - Transfer roasted vegetables to a pot, add vegetable broth, and bring to boil
 - Simmer for 15 min
 - Blend until smooth, stir in apple cider vinegar, black pepper, and coconut cream
 - Garnish with dill fronds
TIPS: Garnish with orange zest for a fragrant note
 - Serve chilled in summer for a refreshing twist
NUTRITIONAL VALUES: Calories: 130 - Fat: 5g - Carbs: 20g - Protein: 2g - Sugar: 12g

BUTTERNUT SQUASH AND SAGE SOUP

PT: 20 min - **CT:** 50 min

MODE: Roasting and Simmering - **SERVS:** 6

INGREDIENTS: 1 medium butternut squash, peeled and cubed

- 3 Tbls olive oil
- 1 onion, diced
- 2 cloves garlic, minced
- 6 sage leaves
- 4 C. chicken bone broth
- 1/2 tsp nutmeg
- Salt and pepper to taste
- 1/4 C. almond milk
- Pumpkin seeds for garnish

DIRECTIONS: Toss butternut squash with 2 Tbls olive oil and roast at 375°F (190°C) for 30 min

- Heat remaining olive oil in a pot
- Add onion, garlic, and sage leaves, cook for 5 min
- Add roasted squash, bone broth, and nutmeg
- Season with salt and pepper
- Simmer for 20 min
- Blend until smooth, stir in almond milk
- Garnish with pumpkin seeds

TIPS: Roast the squash until caramelized for added sweetness

- Swirl with a touch of coconut milk for extra creaminess
- Top with crumbled feta for a tangy contrast

NUTRITIONAL VALUES: Calories: 140 - Fat: 5g - Carbs: 21g - Protein: 3g - Sugar: 6g

FIRE-ROASTED TOMATO AND QUINOA SOUP

PT: 10 min - **CT:** 20 min

MODE: Simmering - **SERVS:** 6

INGREDIENTS: 2 C. fire-roasted tomatoes, canned

- 1 C. quinoa, rinsed
- 1 Tbls coconut oil
- 1 qt. organic chicken stock
- 1 tsp smoked paprika
- 1 tsp dried oregano
- 1 cup spinach, chopped
- Sea salt to taste
- Crushed red pepper flakes for garnish

DIRECTIONS: Heat coconut oil in a soup pot over medium heat

- Add quinoa and toast for 2 min
- Pour in chicken stock and bring to boil
- Stir in fire-roasted tomatoes, smoked paprika, and oregano
- Reduce heat and simmer for 15 min until quinoa is cooked
- Season with sea salt and fold in spinach
- Serve garnished with red pepper flakes

TIPS: Garnish with grated Parmesan cheese for a savory touch

- Add a spoonful of pesto for a flavor twist
- Incorporate a handful of chickpeas for added protein

NUTRITIONAL VALUES: Calories: 160 - Fat: 4g - Carbs: 25g - Protein: 5g - Sugar: 3g

HEARTY TURMERIC LENTIL STEW

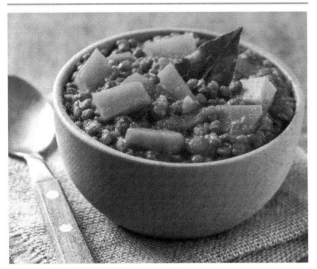

PT: 15 min. - **CT:** 40 min.
MODE: Stovetop - **SERVS:** 6
INGREDIENTS: 1 Tbls extra virgin olive oil

 - 1 med. onion, finely chopped
 - 2 cloves garlic, minced
 - 1 Tbls grated fresh turmeric root
 - 1 tsp ground cumin
 - 2 C. red lentils, rinsed
 - 6 C. low-sodium vegetable broth
 - 1 C. kale, chopped
 - 1 C. butternut squash, cubed
 - 1 Tbls apple cider vinegar
 - Sea salt to taste
 - Freshly ground black pepper to taste

DIRECTIONS: Heat olive oil in a large pot over medium heat

 - Sauté onion until translucent; add garlic, turmeric, and cumin, stirring for 1 min.
 - Add lentils and broth, bring to a simmer, cover, and cook until lentils are tender
 - Add kale and squash, simmer until squash is tender
 - Stir in apple cider vinegar, season with salt and pepper

TIPS: Serve with a squeeze of lemon for a vitamin C boost

 - Top with pumpkin seeds for added crunch and zinc

NUTRITIONAL VALUES: Calories: 250
 - Fat: 3g - Carbs: 42g - Protein: 18g - Sugar: 4g

CREAMY CAULIFLOWER AND LEEK SOUP

PT: 15 min - **CT:** 40 min
MODE: Stovetop - **SERVS:** 4
INGREDIENTS: 1 Tbls butter

 - 1 large leek, sliced and rinsed
 - 1 head cauliflower, chopped
 - 4 C. vegetable broth
 - 1/2 C. heavy cream
 - Salt and pepper to taste
 - Nutmeg for seasoning
 - Chopped chives for garnish

DIRECTIONS: Melt butter in a pot

 - Sauté leek until soft
 - Add cauliflower and broth, bring to a boil then simmer for 30 min
 - Blend until smooth
 - Stir in cream, season with salt, pepper, and nutmeg
 - Serve garnished with chives

TIPS: Garnish with roasted pumpkin seeds for a crunchy texture

 - Substitute heavy cream with coconut milk for a dairy-free version

NUTRITIONAL VALUES: Calories: 220
 - Fat: 16g - Carbs: 16g - Protein: 5g - Sugar: 7g

Miso Mushroom Soup with Silken Tofu

PT: 10 min. - **CT:** 25 min.
MODE: Stovetop - **SERVS:** 4
INGREDIENTS: 4 C. dashi stock

- 2 Tbls miso paste, preferably white
- 1 C. shiitake mushrooms, sliced
- 1 block silken tofu, cubed
- 2 scallions, thinly sliced
- 1 Tbls tamari or soy sauce
- 1 tsp grated ginger root
- 1 Tbls seaweed, chopped, such as wakame or nori

DIRECTIONS: Heat dashi stock in a pot over medium heat

- Dissolve miso paste in a small amount of warm stock and add back to the pot
- Add shiitake mushrooms and simmer for 20 min.
- Add tofu, scallions, tamari, and ginger, heating gently for 5 min.
- Stir in seaweed before serving

TIPS: Avoid boiling as this will destroy beneficial probiotics in miso

- Can be served with a side of steamed brown rice for added fiber

NUTRITIONAL VALUES: Calories: 80 - Fat: 2g - Carbs: 8g - Protein: 6g - Sugar: 2g

Caribbean Curried Sweet Potato Soup

PT: 15 min. - **CT:** 30 min.
MODE: Stovetop - **SERVS:** 6
INGREDIENTS: 1 Tbls coconut oil

- 1 lg. sweet potato, peeled and cubed
- 1 med. carrot, peeled and chopped
- 1 sm. red bell pepper, chopped
- 1 med. onion, chopped
- 3 cloves garlic, minced
- 2 tsp curry powder
- 4 C. low-sodium vegetable broth
- 1 can coconut milk, light
- 1 Tbls fresh lime juice
- Sea salt to taste
- Fresh cilantro for garnish

DIRECTIONS: In a large pot, heat coconut oil over medium heat

- Sauté sweet potato, carrot, bell pepper, and onion until softened
- Add garlic and curry powder, cook for an additional 2 min.
- Pour in broth and bring to a simmer until vegetables are tender
- Blend until smooth, return to pot, and stir in coconut milk and lime juice
- Heat through, and season with salt

TIPS: Garnish with cilantro and a dash of chili flakes for a warm heat

- To add protein, consider topping with roasted chickpeas

NUTRITIONAL VALUES: Calories: 220 - Fat: 6g - Carbs: 38g - Protein: 4g - Sugar: 7g

Roasted Garlic and Cauliflower Soup

PT: 10 min. - **CT:** 45 min.
MODE: Oven and Stovetop - **SERVS:** 4
INGREDIENTS: 1 lg. head of cauliflower, cut into florets

- 3 Tbls extra virgin olive oil
- 1 bulb garlic, top sliced off
- 1 med. onion, diced
- 4 C. low-sodium chicken broth
- 1 tsp dried thyme
- 1 tsp smoked paprika

- Sea salt to taste
- Freshly ground black pepper to taste

DIRECTIONS: Preheat oven to 400°F (200°C)

- Toss cauliflower florets with 2 Tbls olive oil, spread on a baking sheet alongside garlic bulb, and roast for 30 min.
- Squeeze roasted garlic cloves out of their skins and set aside
- Heat remaining oil in a pot and sauté onion
- Add roasted cauliflower, garlic, broth, thyme, and paprika, bringing to a simmer for 15 min.
- Blend until creamy and season with salt and pepper

TIPS: Roasting cauliflower with other vegetables like parsnips adds depth

- Serve with a swirl of cashew cream for a dairy-free richness

NUTRITIONAL VALUES: Calories: 180
- Fat: 11g - Carbs: 17g - Protein: 6g - Sugar: 5g

LEMONGRASS COCONUT SOUP WITH SHRIMP

PT: 10 min. - **CT:** 20 min.
MODE: Stovetop - **SERVS:** 4
INGREDIENTS: 1 Tbls coconut oil

- 2 stalks lemongrass, tender inner parts finely chopped
- 1 C. shiitake mushrooms, sliced
- 1 bell pepper, thinly sliced
- 4 C. low-sodium chicken broth
- 1 lb. shrimp, peeled and deveined
- 1 can coconut milk, light
- 1 Tbls fish sauce
- 2 Tbls lime juice
- 1 Tbls raw honey
- 1 chili pepper, thinly sliced
- Fresh basil for garnish

DIRECTIONS: Heat coconut oil in a large pot over medium heat

- Sauté lemongrass, mushrooms, and bell pepper until aromatic
- Add broth, coconut milk, and fish sauce, bringing to a simmer
- Add shrimp and simmer just until cooked through
- Stir in lime juice and honey, and garnish with chili pepper and basil

TIPS: Infuse soup with kefir lime leaves for added citrus aroma

- Adjust the level of spiciness by increasing or reducing the amount of chili pepper

NUTRITIONAL VALUES: Calories: 270
- Fat: 13g - Carbs: 15g - Protein: 25g - Sugar: 6g

ROASTED RED PEPPER AND TOMATO BISQUE

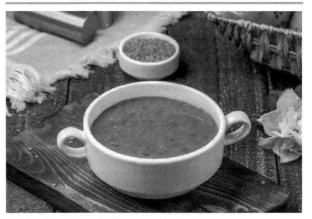

PT: 15 min - **CT:** 30 min
MODE: Stovetop - **SERVS:** 4
INGREDIENTS: 2 Tbls olive oil

- 1 medium onion, chopped
- 2 garlic cloves, minced
- 4 red bell peppers, roasted and peeled
- 4 ripe tomatoes, chopped
- 2 C. vegetable broth

- 1/2 C. almond milk
- Salt and pepper to taste
- Fresh basil leaves for garnish

DIRECTIONS: Heat olive oil in a large pot
- Sauté onion and garlic until translucent
- Add roasted peppers, tomatoes, and broth, bring to a boil then simmer for 20 min
- Blend until smooth
- Stir in almond milk, season with salt and pepper
- Serve garnished with basil leaves

TIPS: Add a pinch of smoked paprika for a smoky flavor
- Can be served with a dollop of cashew cream for richness

NUTRITIONAL VALUES: Calories: 160 - Fat: 7g - Carbs: 23g - Protein: 4g - Sugar: 12g

SPICED RED BELL PEPPER AND TOMATO BISQUE

PT: 15 min. - **CT:** 30 min.
MODE: Stovetop - **SERVS:** 4
INGREDIENTS: 2 Tbls extra virgin olive oil
- 1 med. red bell pepper, chopped
- 1 med. onion, chopped
- 3 cloves garlic, minced
- 2 C. fresh tomatoes, diced
- 2 tsp paprika
- 1 tsp ground coriander
- 4 C. low-sodium vegetable broth
- 2 Tbls tomato paste
- Fresh basil leaves for garnish
- Raw pumpkin seeds for garnish
- Sea salt to taste
- Freshly ground black pepper to taste

DIRECTIONS: Heat olive oil in a pot over medium heat
- Cook bell pepper, onion, and garlic until tender
- Add tomatoes, paprika, coriander, and cook for 2 min.
- Pour in broth, add tomato paste, and simmer for 20 min.
- Blend until smooth and season with salt and pepper

TIPS: Garnish with torn basil leaves and sprinkle with pumpkin seeds
- For an extra creamy texture, blend in a touch of oat milk

NUTRITIONAL VALUES: Calories: 130 - Fat: 7g - Carbs: 15g - Protein: 3g - Sugar: 9g

NORDIC BEETROOT SOUP WITH APPLE

PT: 20 min. - **CT:** 35 min.
MODE: Stovetop - **SERVS:** 4
INGREDIENTS: 2 Tbls extra virgin olive oil
- 4 lg. beetroot, peeled and grated
- 1 lg. apple, peeled and grated
- 1 leek, washed and sliced
- 4 C. low-sodium vegetable broth
- 2 Tbls apple cider vinegar
- 1 tsp caraway seeds
- Sea salt to taste
- Freshly ground black pepper to taste
- 1 dollop dairy-free sour cream for garnish

DIRECTIONS: Heat olive oil in a large pot over medium heat
- Sauté beetroot, apple, and leek for 10 min.
- Add broth and bring to a simmer, cooking until beets are tender
- Stir in apple cider vinegar and caraway seeds and cook for an additional 5 min.

- Season with salt and pepper

TIPS: Serve with a dollop of dairy-free sour cream and a sprinkle of chives

- Enhance the soup with a spoonful of horseradish for zest

NUTRITIONAL VALUES: Calories: 150 - Fat: 7g - Carbs: 20g - Protein: 4g - Sugar: 14g

CHILLED AVOCADO-CUCUMBER SOUP

PT: 10 min - **CT:** 0 min
MODE: No Cooking - **SERVS:** 2
INGREDIENTS: 2 ripe avocados, peeled and pitted

- 1 large cucumber, peeled and chopped
- 1 small jalapeño, seeded and chopped
- 2 cups cold water
- Juice of 1 lime
- 1/2 C. fresh cilantro
- 1 garlic clove
- Salt to taste
- 1/4 C. plain Greek yogurt
- Cucumber slices and cilantro leaves for garnish

DIRECTIONS: Blend avocados, cucumber, jalapeño, water, lime juice, cilantro, and garlic until smooth

- Season with salt
- Stir in yogurt
- Chill in the refrigerator for at least 1 hr
- Serve garnished with cucumber slices and cilantro leaves

TIPS: Serve with toasted whole-grain bread for added texture

- Can be stored in the refrigerator for up to 2 days

NUTRITIONAL VALUES: Calories: 280 - Fat: 20g - Carbs: 24g - Protein: 6g - Sugar: 5g

MISO MUSHROOM BROTH

PT: 10 min - **CT:** 20 min
MODE: Stovetop - **SERVS:** 4
INGREDIENTS: 4 C. vegetable broth

- 1 Tbls miso paste
- 1 Tbls soy sauce
- 2 tsp sesame oil
- 1 C. shiitake mushrooms, sliced
- 1/2 C. tofu, cubed
- 2 green onions, chopped
- 1 Tbls grated ginger
- 1 garlic clove, minced
- Fresh coriander for garnish

DIRECTIONS: Heat broth in a pot over medium heat

- Dissolve miso paste in a small amount of warm broth, add back to the pot
- Add soy sauce, sesame oil, mushrooms, tofu, green onions, ginger, and garlic, simmer for 15 min
- Serve garnished with fresh coriander

TIPS: Add a splash of rice vinegar for a tangy flavor

- Garnish with seaweed strips for extra umami

NUTRITIONAL VALUES: Calories: 120 - Fat: 4g - Carbs: 16g - Protein: 7g - Sugar: 4g

CARROT GINGER SOUP WITH COCONUT AND LEMONGRASS

PT: 10 min - **CT:** 30 min
MODE: Stovetop - **SERVS:** 4
INGREDIENTS: 1 Tbls coconut oil

- 1 lb carrots, peeled and chopped
- 1 Tbls fresh ginger, minced
- 1 stalk lemongrass, minced
- 4 C. vegetable broth

- 1 C. coconut milk
- Salt to taste
- 1 Tbls lemon juice
- Fresh parsley for garnish

DIRECTIONS: Heat coconut oil in a pot

- Sauté carrots, ginger, and lemongrass until fragrant
- Add broth and coconut milk, bring to a boil then simmer for 25 min
- Blend until smooth
- Season with salt and lemon juice
- Serve garnished with parsley

TIPS: Serve with a sprinkle of toasted coconut flakes

- Add a teaspoon of honey for a hint of sweetness

NUTRITIONAL VALUES: Calories: 210 - Fat: 12g - Carbs: 24g - Protein: 3g - Sugar: 8g

SPICY BLACK BEAN SOUP

PT: 15 min - **CT:** 1 hr
MODE: Stovetop - **SERVS:** 6
INGREDIENTS: 1 Tbls olive oil

- 1 large onion, diced
- 2 garlic cloves, minced
- 2 tsp ground cumin
- 1 tsp chili powder
- 4 C. vegetable broth
- 3 C. cooked black beans
- 1 C. diced tomatoes
- Salt and pepper to taste
- Fresh cilantro and lime wedges for garnish

DIRECTIONS: Heat olive oil in a large pot

- Sauté onion and garlic until soft
- Stir in cumin and chili powder
- Add broth, black beans, and tomatoes, bring to a boil then simmer for 45 min
- Season with salt and pepper
- Serve garnished with cilantro and lime wedges

TIPS: Serve with a slice of avocado on top

- Add a splash of hot sauce for extra heat

NUTRITIONAL VALUES: Calories: 190 - Fat: 3g - Carbs: 34g - Protein: 11g - Sugar: 3g

HEALTHY DESSERTS RECIPES

Indulge in the sweet simplicity of desserts that do more than just satisfy your cravings. This chapter is a trove of delectable treats, each crafted to support an anti-inflammatory lifestyle. From ripe, juicy fruits to rich, antioxidant-packed chocolates, we've harnessed nature's bounty to bring you desserts that not only delight your palate but also nourish your body. Embrace a world where every spoonful is a step towards better health.

CHERRY CHIA CELEBRATION PARFAIT

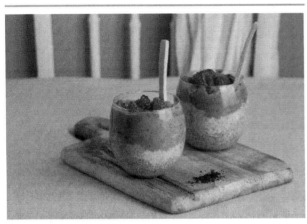

PT: 15 min - **CT:** 0 min
MODE: No Cooking - **SERVS:** 6
INGREDIENTS: 1 C. frozen cherries

- 2 C. Greek yogurt, unsweetened
- ¼ C. chia seeds
- 3 Tbls honey
- ½ tsp almond extract
- 6 Tbls slivered almonds, toasted
- 6 sprigs fresh mint for garnish

DIRECTIONS: Blend frozen cherries, honey, and almond extract until smooth

- In a separate bowl, mix Greek yogurt with chia seeds, let sit for 10 min
- Layer cherry mixture and chia yogurt in glasses
- Top with toasted almonds and mint

TIPS: Garnish with dark chocolate shavings for added antioxidants

- Parfait can be prepped the night before for a richer texture

NUTRITIONAL VALUES: Calories: 180
- Fat: 6g - Carbs: 20g - Protein: 12g - Sugar: 15g

AVOCADO LIME FREEZE

PT: 20 min - **CT:** 2 hr
MODE: Freezing - **SERVS:** 4
INGREDIENTS: 2 ripe avocados

- 1 ripe banana
- Juice of 2 limes
- Zest of 1 lime
- 3 Tbls agave nectar
- 1 C. coconut milk
- 1 tsp vanilla extract
- Pinch of salt

DIRECTIONS: Puree avocados, banana, lime juice, lime zest, agave, coconut milk, vanilla extract, and salt until smooth

- Pour into a loaf pan
- Freeze until solid, about 2 hr
- Scoop and serve

TIPS: Serve with a drizzle of coconut cream for a luxurious touch

- Stir mixture every 30 min while freezing for a smoother texture

NUTRITIONAL VALUES: Calories: 230
- Fat: 15g - Carbs: 25g - Protein: 2g - Sugar: 12g

GINGER-POACHED PEARS

PT: 10 min - **CT:** 25 min
MODE: Poaching - **SERVS:** 4
INGREDIENTS: 4 firm pears, peeled and cored

- 4 C. water
- 1 C. raw honey
- 2 cinnamon sticks
- 1 vanilla bean, split and scraped
- 1 inch ginger root, sliced
- Zest of 1 orange

DIRECTIONS: Combine water, raw honey, cinnamon sticks, vanilla bean, ginger, and orange zest in a saucepan and bring to a simmer

- Add pears and poach until tender
- Remove pears and reduce the liquid to a syrup
- Pour syrup over pears before serving

TIPS: Poaching liquid can be used as a sweetener for teas

- Serve with a dollop of coconut cream

NUTRITIONAL VALUES: Calories: 280
- Fat: 0g - Carbs: 74g - Protein: 1g - Sugar: 70g

SPICED QUINOA APPLE CRISP

PT: 15 min - **CT:** 30 min
MODE: Baking - **SERVS:** 6
INGREDIENTS: Preheat oven to 375°F (190°C)

- 3 C. cooked quinoa
- 4 apples, diced
- ½ C. cranberries, dried
- 1 tsp cinnamon
- ½ tsp nutmeg
- ¼ C. almond flour
- ¼ C. quinoa flakes
- 3 Tbls coconut oil, melted
- 2 Tbls maple syrup

DIRECTIONS: Mix diced apples with cranberries, cinnamon, and nutmeg and place in a baking dish

- Combine almond flour, quinoa flakes, melted coconut oil, and maple syrup for the topping
- Sprinkle over apple mixture
- Bake until golden

TIPS: Top with a sprinkle of hemp seeds for extra crunch and nutrition

- Can be served with unsweetened almond milk custard

NUTRITIONAL VALUES: Calories: 220
- Fat: 8g - Carbs: 34g - Protein: 4g - Sugar: 15g

TURMERIC MANGO MOUSSE

PT: 20 min - **CT:** 1 hr
MODE: Chilling - **SERVS:** 4
INGREDIENTS: 2 C. mango chunks

- 1 tsp turmeric powder
- Juice of 1 lime
- 1 Tbls honey
- 1 can full-fat coconut milk, chilled overnight
- 1 Tbls gelatin powder, dissolved in ¼ C. water
- Mint leaves for garnish

DIRECTIONS: Blend mango chunks, turmeric powder, lime juice, and honey until smooth

- Scoop out the solid coconut cream from the can and whip to soft peaks
- Fold mango mixture into coconut cream
- Add dissolved gelatin
- Chill for 1 hr

TIPS: Garnish with mint leaves and toasted coconut flakes for a refreshing finish

- Gelatin can be replaced with agar powder for a vegetarian option

NUTRITIONAL VALUES: Calories: 210 - Fat: 14g - Carbs: 22g - Protein: 2g - Sugar: 18g

ROASTED BEETROOT AND CHOCOLATE CAKE

PT: 30 min - **CT:** 45 min
MODE: Baking - **SERVS:** 8
INGREDIENTS: Preheat oven to 350°F (175°C)

- 2 medium beetroots, roasted and puréed
- 1 ½ C. almond flour
- ¾ C. raw cacao powder
- 1 tsp baking soda
- ½ tsp sea salt
- 4 large eggs
- ½ C. coconut oil, melted
- ½ C. maple syrup
- 2 tsp vanilla extract

DIRECTIONS: Whisk together almond flour, cacao powder, baking soda, and sea salt

- Beat eggs and mix with beetroot purée, coconut oil, maple syrup, and vanilla
- Combine dry and wet ingredients
- Bake in a lined cake pan until a toothpick comes out clean

TIPS: Serve with a dollop of cashew cream flavored with orange zest

- Use beetroot greens in a salad to accompany the dessert

NUTRITIONAL VALUES: Calories: 320 - Fat: 22g - Carbs: 28g - Protein: 8g - Sugar: 16g

SWEET POTATO PECAN BITES

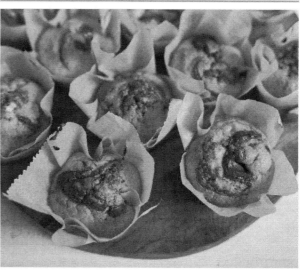

PT: 20 min - **CT:** 0 min
MODE: No Cooking - **SERVS:** 20
INGREDIENTS: 2 medium sweet potatoes, cooked and mashed

- 1 C. pecans, toasted and chopped
- ½ C. medjool dates, pitted
- ¼ tsp ground cloves
- ½ tsp ground ginger
- ½ tsp ground cinnamon
- Shredded coconut for coating

DIRECTIONS: Blend sweet potatoes, pecans, dates, cloves, ginger, and cinnamon until mixture forms a dough

- Roll into bite-sized balls
- Coat with shredded coconut

TIPS: Freeze for 20 min for a firmer texture

- Roll in cocoa powder for a chocolatey version

NUTRITIONAL VALUES: Calories: 100 - Fat: 5g - Carbs: 13g - Protein: 1g - Sugar: 9g

CACAO AND BLUEBERRY FROZEN BARK

PT: 15 min - **CT:** 2 hr
MODE: Freezing - **SERVS:** 12

INGREDIENTS: 2 C. dark chocolate chips, 70% cacao

- 1 C. blueberries, fresh
- ½ C. almonds, chopped
- ½ C. pumpkin seeds
- 1 Tbls coconut oil
- A pinch of fleur de sel

DIRECTIONS: Melt dark chocolate chips with coconut oil

- Pour onto a parchment-lined baking sheet
- Sprinkle with blueberries, almonds, and pumpkin seeds
- Freeze until set
- Break into shards

TIPS: Sprinkle fleur de sel on top before freezing for a gourmet touch

- Use a mix of berries for a variation in flavor and antioxidants

NUTRITIONAL VALUES: Calories: 190 - Fat: 14g - Carbs: 16g - Protein: 4g - Sugar: 12g

GOLDEN TURMERIC CHIA PUDDING

PT: 15 min - **CT:** 0 min
MODE: No Cooking - **SERVS:** 4
INGREDIENTS: 2 C. almond milk

- 1/2 C. chia seeds
- 1/4 C. maple syrup
- 1 tsp vanilla extract
- 1 tsp ground turmeric
- 1/2 tsp ground cinnamon
- Pinch of black pepper
- Fresh mango chunks for topping

DIRECTIONS: Combine almond milk, chia seeds, maple syrup, vanilla extract, ground turmeric, ground cinnamon, and black pepper in a bowl, stirring until homogenous

- Cover and refrigerate overnight or at least 4 hr to let it thicken
- Serve topped with fresh mango chunks

TIPS: Add a dollop of coconut yogurt for creaminess

- Incorporate a sprinkle of bee pollen for an extra boost of anti-inflammatory benefits

NUTRITIONAL VALUES: Calories: 210 - Fat: 9g - Carbs: 29g - Protein: 5g - Sugar: 14g

SPICED PEAR SORBET

PT: 20 min - **CT:** 0 min
MODE: Freezing - **SERVS:** 6
INGREDIENTS: 4 ripe pears, peeled and cored

- 1/2 C. water
- 1 Tbls lemon juice
- 1/4 C. honey
- 1 tsp fresh ginger, grated
- 1/4 tsp ground cardamom
- 1/8 tsp ground nutmeg
- Mint leaves for garnish

DIRECTIONS: Blend pears, water, lemon juice, honey, grated ginger, cardamom, and nutmeg until smooth

- Pour mixture into a shallow pan and freeze until set, about 4-5 hr
- Break frozen mixture into chunks and blend again until smooth and creamy
- Freeze again until ready to serve, garnished with mint leaves

TIPS: Serve immediately after the second blending for a softer texture

- Pair with a drizzle of raw honey for added sweetness

NUTRITIONAL VALUES: Calories: 120 - Fat: 0g - Carbs: 31g - Protein: 0g - Sugar: 25g

ROASTED BALSAMIC FIGS WITH CASHEW CREAM

PT: 15 min - **CT:** 15 min
MODE: Baking - **SERVS:** 4
INGREDIENTS: 8 fresh figs, halved

 - 2 Tbls balsamic vinegar

 - 1 Tbls extra virgin olive oil

 - 1/4 C. raw cashews, soaked for 4 hr

 - 1/4 C. water

 - 1 tsp pure vanilla extract

 - Mint sprigs for garnish

DIRECTIONS: Preheat oven to 350°F (175°C)

 - Toss figs with balsamic vinegar and olive oil, then arrange on a baking sheet cut side up

 - Roast for 15 min

 - While figs are roasting, blend soaked cashews, water, and vanilla extract until smooth to make cashew cream

 - Serve figs with a dollop of cashew cream and garnish with mint sprigs

TIPS: Try drizzling with a touch of organic honey for extra flavor

 - Ensure figs are just ripe for a balance of natural sweetness and texture

NUTRITIONAL VALUES: Calories: 180 - Fat: 8g - Carbs: 27g - Protein: 3g - Sugar: 19g

AVOCADO-CACAO MOUSSE

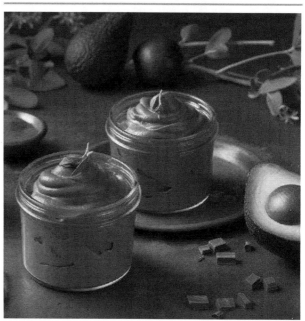

PT: 10 min - **CT:** 0 min
MODE: Blending - **SERVS:** 2
INGREDIENTS: 1 ripe avocado

 - 2 Tbls raw cacao powder

 - 1/4 C. coconut milk

 - 2 Tbls pure maple syrup

 - 1/2 tsp pure vanilla extract

 - A pinch of sea salt

 - Cacao nibs for topping

DIRECTIONS: Blend avocado, raw cacao powder, coconut milk, maple syrup, vanilla extract, and sea salt until smooth

 - Chill for at least 1 hr before serving

 - Top with cacao nibs before serving

TIPS: Add a dash of cinnamon or a drop of peppermint extract for a flavor twist

 - If a thinner consistency is desired, adjust by adding more coconut milk

NUTRITIONAL VALUES: Calories: 345 - Fat: 25g - Carbs: 30g - Protein: 4g - Sugar: 12g

COCONUT-PUMPKIN SEED BRITTLE

PT: 10 min - **CT:** 15 min
MODE: Caramelizing - **SERVS:** 6
INGREDIENTS: 1/2 C. pumpkin seeds, unsalted

- 1 C. coconut sugar
- 1/4 C. water
- 2 Tbls coconut oil
- 1/2 tsp vanilla extract
- Pinch of Himalayan pink salt

DIRECTIONS: Combine coconut sugar and water in a saucepan over medium heat until sugar dissolves

- Increase heat and bring to a boil without stirring until the mixture reaches the hard crack stage, 300°F (149°C), about 15 min
- Remove from heat and swiftly stir in pumpkin seeds, coconut oil, vanilla, and salt
- Pour onto a baking sheet lined with parchment to cool
- Break into pieces once hardened

TIPS: Brush a thin layer of coconut oil on parchment for easy removal

- Store in an airtight container to retain the crunch

NUTRITIONAL VALUES: Calories: 234
- Fat: 14g - Carbs: 25g - Protein: 3g - Sugar: 22g

BERRY QUINOA CRUMBLE

PT: 15 min - **CT:** 30 min
MODE: Baking - **SERVS:** 6
INGREDIENTS: 2 C. mixed berries

- 1 C. quinoa, cooked and cooled
- 1/2 C. almond flour
- 1/4 C. rolled oats
- 1/4 C. walnuts, chopped
- 1/4 C. coconut oil, melted
- 1/4 C. maple syrup
- 1 tsp vanilla extract
- 1/2 tsp ground cinnamon
- A pinch of ground cloves

DIRECTIONS: Preheat oven to 375°F (190°C)

- In a baking dish, layer mixed berries at the bottom
- Toss cooked quinoa with almond flour, rolled oats, chopped walnuts, coconut oil, maple syrup, vanilla extract, ground cinnamon, and cloves until combined
- Spread mixture over berries
- Bake for 30 min or until topping is golden

TIPS: Serve with a dollop of coconut cream for added luxury

- Use a mixture of frozen and fresh berries for varied texture and flavor

NUTRITIONAL VALUES: Calories: 285
- Fat: 15g - Carbs: 35g - Protein: 5g - Sugar: 12g

CHILLED LIME AVOCADO TART

PT: 25 min - **CT:** 2 hr
MODE: Chilling - **SERVS:** 8
INGREDIENTS: 2 ripe avocados

- 1/2 C. raw cashews, soaked overnight
- 1 C. almond flour
- 1 C. pitted dates, soaked for 30 min
- 1/4 C. coconut oil, melted
- Zest and juice of 2 limes
- 1/4 C. pure maple syrup
- Sea salt to taste

DIRECTIONS: Process almond flour and soaked dates in a food processor until it forms a sticky dough

- Press dough into the base of a tart tin and chill to set

- Blend avocados, soaked cashews, coconut oil, lime zest and juice, maple syrup, and sea salt until creamy

- Pour over crust and chill for at least 2 hr

TIPS: Garnish with lime slices and zest for a refreshing twist

- Add a touch of spirulina for a brighter green color

NUTRITIONAL VALUES: Calories: 320 - Fat: 22g - Carbs: 29g - Protein: 5g - Sugar: 15g

CHAI-SPICED BAKED PEARS

PT: 15 min. - **CT:** 25 min.
MODE: Baking - **SERVS:** 4
INGREDIENTS: 4 ripe but firm pears, halved and cored

- 2 Tbls raw honey

- 1 tsp ground cinnamon

- ¼ tsp ground ginger

- ⅛ tsp ground cloves

- ⅛ tsp ground cardamom

- 1 Tbls coconut oil, melted

- 1 C. almond flour

- 2 Tbls chopped walnuts

DIRECTIONS: Stir together honey, cinnamon, ginger, cloves, and cardamom in a small bowl

- Brush this mixture over the cut side of pears

- Place pears cut side up in a baking dish

- Combine melted coconut oil and almond flour until mixture resembles coarse crumbs

- Sprinkle this topping and walnuts over pears

- Bake in preheated oven at 350°F (175°C) until pears are tender

TIPS: Serve with a dollop of coconut cream to add a creamy texture

- Walnuts can be substituted with pecans for a different flavor profile

NUTRITIONAL VALUES: Calories: 210 - Fat: 9g - Carbs: 32g - Protein: 3g - Sugar: 23g

GINGER ZUCCHINI BREAD

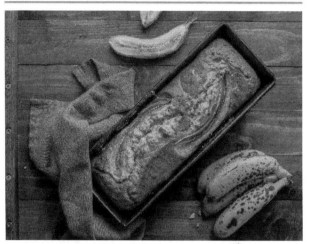

PT: 10 min - **CT:** 50 min
MODE: Baking - **SERVS:** 8
INGREDIENTS: 1 1/2 C. whole wheat flour

- 1/2 tsp baking soda

- 1/2 tsp baking powder

- 1/4 tsp sea salt

- 1 Tbls ground ginger

- 1/4 C. apple sauce, unsweetened

- 1/4 C. olive oil

- 1/4 C. almond milk

- 1/2 C. zucchini, finely grated

- 1/4 C. pure maple syrup

- 1/2 tsp almond extract

DIRECTIONS: Preheat oven to 350°F (175°C)

- Mix whole wheat flour, baking soda, baking powder, sea salt, and ground ginger in a bowl

- In a separate bowl, whisk apple sauce, olive oil, almond milk, grated zucchini, maple syrup, and almond extract

- Combine wet and dry ingredients and pour into a greased loaf pan

- Bake for 50 min or until a toothpick comes out clean

TIPS: Introduce finely chopped crystallized ginger for a vibrant flavor burst

- Allow to cool in pan for 10 min before transferring to a wire rack

NUTRITIONAL VALUES: Calories: 165 - Fat: 9g - Carbs: 20g - Protein: 3g - Sugar: 6g

GINGERED BLUEBERRY SORBET

PT: 10 min. - **CT:** 2 hrs. freezing
MODE: Freezing - **SERVS:** 6
INGREDIENTS: 3 C. frozen blueberries

- ¼ C. raw honey

- Juice of 1 lemon

- 2 tsp freshly grated ginger root

- Fresh mint leaves for garnish

DIRECTIONS: Blend frozen blueberries, raw honey, lemon juice, and grated ginger in a food processor until smooth

- Pour into a freezer-safe container

- Freeze until solid, stirring every 30 min. to break up ice crystals

TIPS: Garnish with fresh mint leaves before serving for a refreshing twist

- Can be made ahead and stored in the freezer for up to 2 weeks

NUTRITIONAL VALUES: Calories: 120 - Fat: 0g - Carbs: 31g - Protein: 1g - Sugar: 27g

AVOCADO LIME CHEESECAKE

PT: 20 min. - **CT:** 4 hrs. chilling
MODE: No Baking - **SERVS:** 8
INGREDIENTS: 2 medium ripe avocados

- 1 C. raw cashews, soaked overnight and drained

- ½ C. coconut cream

- Juice and zest of 2 limes

- ⅓ C. raw honey

- 1 tsp pure vanilla extract

- ½ C. coconut oil, melted

- 1 C. almond flour

- ¼ C. unsweetened shredded coconut

DIRECTIONS: Puree avocados, cashews, coconut cream, lime juice, and zest, raw honey, and vanilla extract until creamy

- Slowly add in the melted coconut oil while continuing to blend

- Press almond flour and shredded coconut into the base of the springform pan to form a crust

- Pour avocado mixture over the crust

- Chill in refrigerator until set

TIPS: For a nut-free option, replace almond flour with oat flour

- The lime zest garnish enhances flavor and aesthetics

NUTRITIONAL VALUES: Calories: 320 - Fat: 28g - Carbs: 20g - Protein: 4g - Sugar: 12g

SPICED PUMPKIN MOUSSE

PT: 15 min. - **CT:** 2 hrs. chilling
MODE: No Cooking - **SERVS:** 6
INGREDIENTS: 1 15-oz. can pumpkin puree

- 1 ½ C. full-fat coconut milk
- ¼ C. raw honey
- 1 tsp ground cinnamon
- ½ tsp ground nutmeg
- ¼ tsp ground ginger
- ⅛ tsp ground cloves
- 1 Tbls gelatin, bloom in ¼ C. water

DIRECTIONS: Whisk together pumpkin puree, coconut milk, raw honey, cinnamon, nutmeg, ginger, and cloves in a large bowl

- Dissolve bloomed gelatin over low heat, then whisk into pumpkin mixture until well combined
- Pour into dessert cups
- Chill until mousse is set

TIPS: Top each serving with a sprinkle of cinnamon or nutmeg for added aroma

- This mousse can be served as a filling for a grain-free tart shell

NUTRITIONAL VALUES: Calories: 200 - Fat: 14g - Carbs: 18g - Protein: 2g - Sugar: 12g

DARK CHOCOLATE ALMOND CLUSTERS

PT: 10 min. - **CT:** 15 min.
MODE: Refrigeration - **SERVS:** 10
INGREDIENTS: 1 ½ C. dark chocolate chips, at least 70% cacao

- 1 C. raw almonds
- 1 Tbls coconut oil
- 1 tsp ground cinnamon
- 1 tsp pure vanilla extract
- Flaky sea salt for sprinkling

DIRECTIONS: Melt dark chocolate chips and coconut oil together in a double boiler, stirring occasionally

- Remove from heat and stir in cinnamon and vanilla extract
- Fold in raw almonds until evenly coated
- Drop spoonfuls of mixture onto a parchment-lined tray
- Sprinkle with flaky sea salt
- Refrigerate until hardened

TIPS: Store leftovers in an airtight container in the refrigerator to maintain texture

- Use a silicone mat for easy removal of clusters

NUTRITIONAL VALUES: Calories: 150 - Fat: 12g - Carbs: 9g - Protein: 3g - Sugar: 6g

COCONUT FLOUR LEMON BARS

PT: 20 min. - **CT:** 22 min.
MODE: Baking - **SERVS:** 9
INGREDIENTS: Crust: 1 C. coconut flour

- ⅓ C. coconut oil, melted
- 2 Tbls raw honey
- 1 Tbls ground flaxseed
- Filling: 4 large eggs
- ½ C. raw honey
- ⅓ C. lemon juice
- 2 tsp lemon zest
- ¼ tsp turmeric
- 1 tsp pure vanilla extract

DIRECTIONS: To make the crust, combine coconut flour, melted coconut oil, raw honey, and ground flaxseed and press into bottom of a greased 8x8-inch baking pan

- Bake at 350°F (175°C) for 10 min. until golden

- Beat eggs, raw honey, lemon juice, lemon zest, turmeric, and vanilla extract until smooth

- Pour over baked crust

- Bake for an additional 12 min. or until filling is set

TIPS: Cut into squares when cool

- Allow bars to chill in the fridge before serving for best texture

- Turmeric adds a boost of anti-inflammatory benefits and a vibrant color

NUTRITIONAL VALUES: Calories: 230 - Fat: 13g - Carbs: 24g - Protein: 5g - Sugar: 18g

5-WEEK MEAL PLAN: YOUR ROADMAP TO SUCCESS

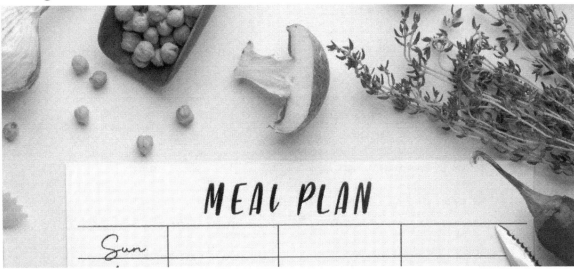

Embarking on a journey to improve your health through diet can often seem like a daunting task, particularly when your days are already brimming with responsibility. But take heart; for it is not the swift sprint but the steadfast march that wins the day. Over the next five weeks, as you weave the principles of anti-inflammatory eating into the intricate tapestry of your daily life, you will discover that each thread of considered choice adds strength and vibrancy to the whole.

Dedicating yourself to this 5-week meal plan is akin to setting sail toward a horizon brimming with vitality and zest. Each week, you'll find a rewarding balance—courses that will brighten the grayest of mornings, salads that jazz up the humdrum lunch, and dinners that turn tables into altars of wellness. And you, at the heart of this transformative experience, will gain not just delicious meals but an education in cultivating lasting well-being.

Week 1: Acquaintance and Adjustment

In the initial week, gently introduce your palate to new flavors. Dedicate this time to exploring the variety of nutrient-dense foods you've stocked in your pantry. Imagine your plate as a painter's palette—splash it with vibrant colors from an array of vegetables, smooth out textures with whole grains, and add depth with lean proteins. You'll start with more familiar dishes, gradually incorporating anti-inflammatory ingredients.

WEEK 1	Sunday	Monday	Tuesday	Wednesday	Thursday	Friday	Saturday
breakfast	Savory Spinach and Sweet Potato Hash	Chia Seed and Coconut Milk Porridge	Anti-Inflammatory Turmeric Scramble	Anti-Inflammatory Blueberry Smoothie Bowl	Mushroom and Kale Frittata Muffins	Buckwheat and Zucchini Pancakes	Ginger-Infused Oatmeal with Poached Pears
snack	Avocado and Edamame Smash	Cumin-Infused Beet Hummus	Sesame Ginger Eggplant Sticks	Spiced Moroccan Carrot Dip	Zesty Lime and Chia Seed Hummus	Charred Shishito Peppers with Lemon Aioli	Sun-Dried Tomato and Olive Tapenade
lunch	Rainbow Chard and Pomegranate Salad	Spicy Roasted Cauliflower with Tahini	Jicama and Orange Citrus Burst Salad	Kale and Avocado Massaged Salad	Charred Broccolini with Lemon Herb Vinaigrette	Roasted Beetroot and Arugula Symphony	Spicy Kale and Quinoa Power Bowl
snack	Cherry Chia Celebration Parfait	Ginger-Poached Pears	Avocado Lime Freeze	Golden Turmeric Chia Pudding	Spiced Pear Sorbet	Coconut-Pumpkin Seed Brittle	Avocado Lime Cheesecake
dinner	Citrus-Infused Salmon Carpaccio	Harissa-Rubbed Grilled Chicken Skewers	Thai-Style Mussels with Lemongrass Broth	Balsamic Fig Chicken Thighs	Cajun Blackened Cod with Mango Avocado Salsa	Poulet à l'Estragon	Seared Scallops with Pomegranate Beurre Blanc

Week 2: Rhythm and Routine

As the sun ushers in the second week, you've begun to embrace the subtle shifts in your routine. Breakfasts brimming with antioxidant-rich berries and oats have replaced the bagel-on-the-go, while lunches are redefined with hearty, leafy salads dotted with nuts and seeds. Dinner becomes a family affair; a time to savor grilled fish or a lean chicken dish as you share the day's experiences.

WEEK 2	Sunday	Monday	Tuesday	Wednesday	Thursday	Friday	Saturday
breakfast	Golden Milk Steel-Cut Oat Risotto	Spirulina & Coconut Porridge	Anti-Inflammatory Blueberry Smoothie Bowl	Cinnamon Quinoa Breakfast Bowl	Shakshuka with Leafy Greens	Avocado and White Bean Toast	Miso-Infused Scrambled Eggs
snack	Balsamic Roasted Carrots	Herb-Infused Mushroom Pâté	Sesame Ginger Bok Choy	Spiced Beet and Lentil Salad	Zesty Lime and Chia Seed Hummus	Crispy Turmeric Cauliflower Florets	Charred Edamame with Sea Salt and Citrus Zest
lunch	Rainbow Radish and Edamame Salad with Ume Plum Dressing	Shaved Brussels Sprout and Manchego Salad	Kohlrabi Slaw with Ginger Lime Dressing	Charred Eggplant with Pomegranate and Tahini Drizzle	Caramelized Fennel and Citrus Crunch	Mizuna and Roasted Root Vegetable Salad	Spicy Kale and Quinoa Power Bowl
snack	Ginger Zucchini Bread	Avocado-Cacao Mousse	Chilled Lime Avocado Tart	Berry Quinoa Crumble	Spiced Pumpkin Mousse	Gingered Blueberry Sorbet	Chai-Spiced Baked Pears
dinner	Grilled Swordfish with Mango Salsa	Pomegranate Glazed Cornish Hen	Cajun-Spiced Catfish with Collard Greens	Harissa-Rubbed Swordfish Steaks	Sesame-Ginger Ground Turkey Stir-Fry	Tarragon-Infused Orange Roughy	Mediterranean Chicken Kabobs

Week 3: Exploration and Experimentation

With a solid two weeks of transformed eating behind you, now is the time to be adventurous with herbs and spices. Let bold blends and exotic flavors transport you to far-off lands. A Moroccan-styled stew for dinner or an Asian fusion salad for lunch could easily become new favorites. This week serves as a nudge to push the culinary envelope and test how these worldly tastes might just become part of your everyday table.

WEEK 3	Sunday	Monday	Tuesday	Wednesday	Thursday	Friday	Saturday
breakfast	Golden Turmeric Yogurt Bowl	Avocado Toast with Tomato and Pumpkin Seeds	Savory Turmeric Oatmeal	Shakshuka with Leafy Greens	Spirulina & Coconut Porridge	Chia and Hemp Seed Parfait	Warm Ginger-Pear Breakfast Salad
snack	Spiced Moroccan Carrot Dip	Curried Cauliflower Florets	Zesty Lime and Chia Seed Hummus	Sesame Ginger Eggplant Sticks	Charred Edamame with Sea Salt and Citrus Zest	Herb-Infused Mushroom Pâté	Spiced Beet and Lentil Salad
lunch	Jicama and Watercress Salad with Citrus Vinaigrette	Charred Broccolini with Tahini Sauce	Spicy Roasted Cauliflower with Tahini	Rainbow Radish and Edamame Salad with Ume Plum Dressing	Kohlrabi Slaw with Ginger Lime Dressing	Shaved Brussels Sprouts with Warm Bacon Vinaigrette	Chilled Zucchini Ribbon Salad with Lemon-Herb Dressing
snack	Coconut-Pumpkin Seed Brittle	Ginger-Poached Pears	Avocado Lime Freeze	Spiced Pear Sorbet	Chai-Spiced Baked Pears	Avocado-Cacao Mousse	Berry Quinoa Crumble
dinner	Moroccan Chicken with Pomegranate and Walnuts (Fesenjan)	Thai-Style Mussels with Lemongrass Broth	Harissa-Rubbed Grilled Chicken Skewers	Miso-Marinated Black Cod	Cioppino with a Twist	Pistachio-Crusted Barramundi with Citrus Aioli	Harissa-Rubbed Swordfish Steaks

Week 4: Fine-Tuning and Feedback

By week four, the effects of your food choices may be whispering—or shouting—their benefits to your body. Take stock of these changes. Are you sleeping better? Have those nagging aches lessened their grip? Your plate is now a familiar friend rather than a foreign concept, and you might find joy in tweaking recipes to suit your tastes even more. Your relationship with food is deepening, evolving—fine-tune it as you would a cherished melody.

WEEK 4	Sunday	Monday	Tuesday	Wednesday	Thursday	Friday	Saturday
breakfast	Miso-Infused Scrambled Eggs	Avocado and White Bean Toast	Buckwheat and Zucchini Pancakes	Chia Seed and Coconut Milk Porridge	Spirulina & Coconut Porridge	Golden Turmeric Yogurt Bowl	Anti-Inflammatory Turmeric Scramble
snack	Sesame Ginger Bok Choy	Spiced Beetroot and Quinoa Tabbouleh	Curried Cauliflower Florets	Charred Edamame with Sea Salt and Citrus Zest	Zesty Lime and Chia Seed Hummus	Balsamic Roasted Carrots	Herb-Infused Mushroom Pâté
lunch	Spicy Kale and Quinoa Power Bowl	Shaved Brussels Sprout and Manchego Salad	Mizuna and Roasted Root Vegetable Salad	Roasted Beetroot and Arugula Symphony	Jicama and Watercress Salad with Citrus Vinaigrette	Rainbow Radish and Edamame Salad with Ume Plum Dressing	Charred Eggplant with Pomegranate and Tahini Drizzle
snack	Gingered Blueberry Sorbet	Chai-Spiced Baked Pears	Coconut-Pumpkin Seed Brittle	Avocado Lime Cheesecake	Spiced Pumpkin Mousse	Spiced Pear Sorbet	Berry Quinoa Crumble
dinner	Pistachio-Crusted Salmon	Turmeric-Ginger Chicken Stir-Fry	Cajun Blackened Cod with Mango Avocado Salsa	Pollo Pibil	Harissa-Roasted Chicken Thighs	Tarragon-Infused Orange Roughy	Maple-Mustard Spatchcock Chicken

Week 5: Reflection and Reinforcement

The final week is about reflection—taking a moment to appreciate the blooming of seeds sown weeks ago. It's also a crucial time to reinforce the practices that will carry forth beyond these 35 days. Keep simplifying, strategizing, and savoring each meal. When choosing a creamy squash soup for its comforting embrace or a crisp apple for its satisfying crunch, you are reaffirming your commitment to this healthier, more vibrant path.

WEEK 5	Sunday	Monday	Tuesday	Wednesday	Thursday	Friday	Saturday
breakfast	Golden Milk Steel-Cut Oat Risotto	Warm Ginger-Pear Breakfast Salad	Chia and Hemp Seed Parfait	Anti-Inflammatory Shakshuka	Avocado Toast with Tomato and Pumpkin Seeds	Miso-Infused Scrambled Eggs	Spirulina & Coconut Porridge
snack	Avocado and Edamame Smash	Sesame Ginger Eggplant Sticks	Curried Cauliflower Florets	Zesty Lime and Chia Seed Hummus	Spiced Beet and Lentil Salad	Charred Shishito Peppers with Lemon Aioli	Balsamic Roasted Carrots
lunch	Warm Spinach and Mushroom Saute	Beetroot Carpaccio with Arugula and Feta	Charred Broccolini with Lemon Herb Vinaigrette	Jicama and Orange Citrus Burst Salad	Rainbow Radish and Edamame Salad with Ume Plum Dressing	Kale and Avocado Massaged Salad	Spicy Kale and Quinoa Power Bowl
snack	Ginger Zucchini Bread	Spiced Quinoa Apple Crisp	Avocado-Cacao Mousse	Coconut-Pumpkin Seed Brittle	Chai-Spiced Baked Pears	Berry Quinoa Crumble	Spiced Pear Sorbet
dinner	Citrus-Infused Grilled Octopus	Harissa-Rubbed Swordfish Steaks	Grilled Scallops with Pomegranate Salsa	Pistachio-Crusted Barramundi with Citrus Aioli	Za'atar Spiced Turkey Cutlets	Mediterranean Chicken Kabobs	Cajun Blackened Cod with Mango Avocado Salsa

Throughout these weeks, keep a few things in mind:

Meals should not be a tyranny of the clock. If an early dinner suits your lifestyle more, adjust the plan accordingly. The key word here is sustainability, finding natural spaces within your day for these nourishing meals.

Portion sizes are whispers, not decrees. Every body speaks in a unique dialect of needs and satisfaction. Listen to yours. Remember, this is not only about what you eat, but also about honoring when you've had enough.

Cooking at home is an art of love. Every chop, stir, and simmer is a brushstroke in a masterpiece you offer to yourself and your loved ones. It's the secret ingredient that makes even the simplest dish sparkle with care.

Flexibility is the sous-chef of life. Change the side dish if the store is out of kale, use frozen berries if fresh are out of season. The plan is your guide, not your guard.

Mindfulness is a companion at the table. Savor each bite, noting not just the taste, but the textures, the colors, the aromas. These are the moments that build a lifetime of healthful habits.

Mainly, remember why you started. You sought to quench inflammation's fires, to nurture your family, to infuse your days with energy. These dishes, they are but the beginning of your journey, not the entirety of it. They are a promise to yourself, plated and presented with care.

As you progress through these five weeks, carry with you the understanding that change is a mosaic of small choices. Each day is a fresh opportunity to build upon the last, and every meal is a chance to fuel your body and spirit in harmonious concert. The beauty of this meal plan is not in its capacity to revolutionize your diet in dramatic sweeps, but in its gentle guidance towards a more mindful, healthful approach to eating—one that will support you for 1500 days and beyond.

CONCLUSION

As we draw the final strokes on our canvas of culinary healing, I am buoyed by the thought that this book may have sparked a gentle yet transformative revolution in your kitchen, and hence, your life. In threading our way through the forest of wholesome ingredients and vibrant recipes, we've laid a foundation for nurturing your body, fortifying your immune system, and embarking on a serene journey toward wellness.

Throughout these pages, we've traversed a landscape rich with possibilities—learning not just to cook, but to cook with purpose, crafting each dish to serve as a stepping stone to greater health. If anything, let us remember that this journey does not culminate with the last page; it is designed to be expansive and forgiving, allowing for improvisation and adaptation to your unique tapestry of needs.

Amid your bustling days, where deadlines loom large and commitments crowd the calendar, you've found the resilience to prioritize your health, understanding that nourishment is not just about satiating hunger but about enriching life. The transformation promised by an anti-inflammatory lifestyle is neither abrupt nor fleeting—it is a testament to the compounded effects of daily choices.

We've ventured together through a mosaic of flavors and textures that, I hope, has dispelled any lingering skepticism about the palatability of healthful cooking. The meals we've shared stand as vibrant proof that nutrition need not come at the cost of taste, and that simplicity, even on a tight budget, can yield gastronomic delight. Remember, your kitchen is more than a place of provision; it is a sanctuary where wellness begins and flourishes.

Embarking on this path may have seemed daunting at first, especially when past attempts at healthier living may have met less than inspiring ends. But with each meal prepared and enjoyed, your confidence has burgeoned, your skills sharpened, and surely your well-being has reaped the benefits. As each day's menu unfolds, let the rich tapestry of flavors remind you of your capacity for change and renewal.

The narratives sprinkled throughout from individuals who, like you, embarked on this journey with trepidation, only to find solace and success, are mirrors reflecting the possibilities that lie ahead. Their stories are woven from threads of challenge and triumph, offering both solace and inspiration to press forward when the path seems steep.

In these times, when information is a steady torrent that threatens to overwhelm rather than enlighten, the simple principles of the anti-inflammatory diet stand as a beacon. Through discernment, we cut through the noise, focusing on the healing properties of whole foods rather than the clamor of dietary fads and unattainable ideals.

What of your children, your partner, your cherished circle of family and friends? This foray into informed eating is a gift to them as well; an inheritance of health and a testament of your love. As they come to relish the nuanced flavors of vegetables, whole grains, and lean proteins, they, too, will grasp the joy of foods that heal rather than harm. An anti-inflammatory lifestyle, after all, is a familial journey—one that promises collective nourishment and joy.

I know that for some, the lure of fast food and the convenience it promises is a potent foil, a temptation always lurking. Yet, as you've trudged through the early days, triumphing over time constraints and counterbalancing culinary doubts, you've proven to yourself that the promise of health is within reach—and well worth the investment of your time and creativity.

Consider this not an end, but a milestone; for learning and growth in the kitchen and in our approach to eating are lifelong pursuits. This book has sought to be your ally, your culinary compass, guiding you to choices that benefit both body and soul, through times of celebration and challenge alike.

Before we part ways, let me leave you with a dollop of encouragement: hold fast to the strides you've made. Know that the road to well-being is rarely a straight path; it meanders, sometimes backtracks, but always leads forward. On days when your resolve wavers, remember why you began—clarity in mind, vitality in body, peace in spirit.

In closing, cherish the communal aspect of meals; savor not just the flavors, but the shared experiences, the laughter, the conversations. These gatherings are the lifeblood of your anti-inflammatory lifestyle, each recipe a verse in your greater story of health.

May your pantry always brim with healing staples, your tables with plates infused with care, and your heart with the satisfaction of nurturing those you hold dear. As you move onward from these instructional shores, may you carry with you the essence of what we've cultivated here—a robust, spirited approach to eating that elevates living to an art.

In gratitude for the trust you've placed in these pages and the journey we've embarked on together, I bid you a heartfelt bon appétit and a vibrant voyage ahead.

A SPECIAL THANK YOU

I hope you found inspiration and insight in the pages of this book. Your journey to health and harmony is important to me, and I'm excited to offer two exclusive, complimentary bonuses to enhance your experience:

"Smoothies to Soothe: Anti-Inflammatory Blends for Health & Harmony" - Discover delicious and nutritious smoothie recipes designed to reduce inflammation and boost your well-being.

"Your Ultimate Anti-Inflammatory Shopping List" - Simplify your grocery runs with a comprehensive list of ingredients that support a healthy, anti-inflammatory lifestyle.

To access these valuable resources, simply scan the QR codes below.

As you embark on this path of health and harmony, I would love to hear about your journey. If you've enjoyed this book and found it helpful, please consider leaving an honest review. Your feedback not only supports me but also helps others discover the benefits of a balanced, anti-inflammatory lifestyle.

Here's to your health!

SMOOTHIES TO SOOTHE

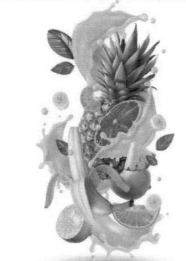

ANTI-INFLAMMATORY BLENDS

FOR HEALTH & HARMONY

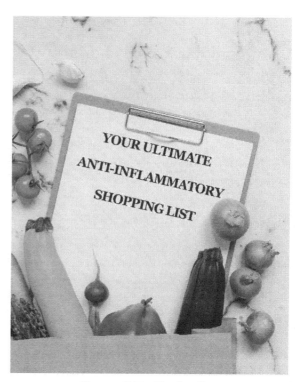

Scan QR Code for
"Smoothies to Soothe"

Scan QR Code for
"Your Ultimate Anti-Inflammatory
Shopping List"

Made in the USA
Middletown, DE
30 October 2024

63568153R00062